THE POWER OF $ELF CARE

A Common Sense Guide to Investing in YOUR Wellness Solution

DR. NANCY GAHLES, DC, CCH, RSHOM(NA)

ISBN-10: 1470013789
EAN-13: 9781470013783

DEDICATION

To my husband, Stewart, who gave me the one thing I couldn't give myself, my two beloved children, Jade and Skylar, and who continues to walk beside me on the path of revelation of unconditional love.

My beloved Jade and Skylar, the shining stars in my firmament, who affirm for me all the goodness in life.

And to my devoted secretary and right hand wonder woman, Erin Green, who has been the steadfast support of my professional life.

TABLE OF CONTENTS

ACKNOWLEDGEMENTS

I gratefully and lovingly acknowledge my parents, George and Pat Gahles, who gave me the spirit of "I can", the enthusiasm for the path of learning, the compassion for care giving, the treasure of family, and very importantly, the gift of laughter.

My siblings, Kathy, Rainy, Patti, Jacquie, G.M. and Timmy, the glue that holds a family together in love and loyalty.

My patients and friends who have graciously allowed me to "practice" on them and taught me volumes on the art of healing.

My colleagues on the Board of Directors of the National Center for Homeopathy for their encouragement, support and active pursuit of educating about and mainstreaming homeopathy.

Finally, two women whose mentoring, courage, and virtues of strength, tenacity, truth and wisdom, taught me to never, never, never give up! Heartfelt gratitude to Sharon Stevenson and Jean Hoagland. Excelsior, ladies!

Photo credit: Brian McCarthy, McCarthyphotostudio.com

Cover design, inspiration and constant encouragement to get this book out: Mr. Lodestar, Lodestar Statements in Stone, www.lodestarstone.com

Charts and graphs: special thanks to Skylar Ritwo

More Praise quotes:

"*The Power of $elf Care* is a great introduction to thinking about and taking action on our health...gives advice on investing in health and on health care spending...and how to rekindle your personal vision." – Clement Bezold, Ph.D., Chairman and Senior Futurist, Institute for Alternative Futures.

"This gift from Dr. Gahles is for everyone. Her insights regarding health, wellness, and self actualization are jewels to be reflected upon and savored". Leonard A. Wisneski, MD, FACP Georgetown University Faculty George Washington University Faculty University of Colorado Faculty.

PREFACE

What is self care?

The new paradigm in healthcare is self care. It is the future of healthcare born of this moment in time. A paradigm is a framework of commonly accepted views on a subject. Self care represents a shift in the prevailing reductionist, hierarchical, patriarchical method of treating disease to one that puts the person/patient at the center, considers the whole person and is inclusive, collaborative and transparent emphasizing personal responsibility and individuality.

The World Health Organization (WHO) defines self care as "activities individuals, families, and communities undertake with the intention of enhancing health, preventing disease, limiting illness, and restoring health. These activities are derived from knowledge and skills from the pool of both professional and lay experience. They are undertaken by lay people on their own behalf, either separately or in participative collaboration with professionals."

Other definitions of self care describe the individual behavior in health promotion and prevention or in disease detection and treatment.

The big idea is that individuals can be active participants in the healthcare of themselves and their families. People are already doing that. With the advent of the Internet and it's vast information highway, many people self diagnose and self treat after looking up symptoms and selecting a treatment that they feel is appropriate for them. Some studies report that 80-95% of health problems are managed at home. Should the problem continue or return, this is when people seek the advice of a medical doctor or other professional. This is as it should be. If we are to manage costs of an already overburdened system of care providing, we need to shift some of the responsibility to the individual who has the problem. The data points to the fact that diabetics, asthmatics and other chronic patients can manage their own care as well as or better than conventional care and at lower costs. NIH studies show that upwards of 38% of Americans are using other systems of medicine to manage their symptoms and to promote health and prevent disease.

Stakeholders in the healthcare industry are calling for a revolution.

So, why is a revolution necessary?

Revolution, derived from the Latin revolutio, means to turn around. A revolution in society is undertaken to make a change in the fundamental or prevailing power or organizational structure. A revolution conjures up the image of war, guns, a battleground. This is usually because the powers that be don't give way to losing their authority so easily. At some point, the people speak and demand the changes they have been asking for. When the critical mass is reached, the people overthrow the existing system in a relatively short period of time.

The revolution that I am speaking about with regard to self care has the seeds of all the revolutions in history. People want their power back. People want the opportunities that education and resources allow for them to become responsible and self sufficient. People no longer want their healthcare to be dictated by the terms of the insurance companies or by government. People no longer want to be obligated to use only one system of medicine when others exist that afford safe, non-toxic, affordable solutions to their healthcare issues. People want to be heard. They want a practitioner who listens to the story of their suffering. They want a practitioner who gets that and whom is knowledgable enough to refer to the practice that will best suit the needs of the whole person. People want choices other than drugs and surgery.

The *NEW* healthcare revolution has all the earmarks of the American Revolution. It is a *WELLNESS* revolution.

Benjamin Rush was a medical doctor and a signer of the Declaration of Independence. He was a social activist and a popular figure at the height of his influence in medicine. He championed freedom in medicine as a human right.

> "Unless we put medical freedom into the Constitution, the time will come when medicine will organize into an undercover dictatorship to restrict the art of healing to one class of Men and deny equal privileges to others; the Constitution of the Republic should make a Special privilege for medical freedoms as well as religious freedom."
> – Benjamin Rush

At this moment in time, we, the people, have the art of healing restricted to one class of Men. In my understanding, this is organized medicine as an undercover dictatorship denying equal privileges to others. This is exactly what Dr. Rush attempted to prevent from happening.

The *WELLNESS* Revolution that I champion is one that will assure the rights of the people to CHOICE and ACCESS to the healthcare systems of their choice.

Doctors are people too. A recent study showed that 50% of medical doctors were dissatisfied with the practice of medicine. Why? Because there is no one answer to every problem that a patient presents with. People are whole complex systems of physical, mental, emotional, spiritual networks that require thought and considerate intervention in order to bring them back into balance. It stands to reason that this cannot be accomplished in every case with pharmaceuticals or technology or surgery. As the old adage says, "if you only have a hammer, everything looks like a nail."

Doctors and their patients are sick of being sick. There is a vast world of care and solutions that can be accessed beyond conventional medicine. Revolutions indeed turn things around. We need a revolution when we have spoken up about the lack of choice and access for years and no one is listening. No one is willing to facilitate change in the system. Why? Because money is being made in the powerful pharmaceutical industry and they have control over the game. The medical doctors are the handmaidens of the medical/industrial complex.

It is clear that change in the fundamental structure is needed, it is clear that those in healthcare circles want it. They are not asking for a total overthrow of the existing system. There are some fine components in drugs and surgery and the technological advancements that save lives in emergencies . What do they want? They want an integrative healthcare system.

What is integrative healthcare?

Integrative healthcare is the practice of healthcare that reaffirms the importance of the relationship between practitioner and patient, focuses on the whole person, is informed by evidence, both researched and clinical real-world outcomes and makes use of all appropriate therapeutic approaches, healthcare professionals and disciplines to achieve optimal health and healing.

In February, 2009, the Institute of Medicine of the National Academies held a Summit on Integrative Medicine and the Health of the Public. The program was to provide a unique opportunity to examine the role and value of integrative medicine in more fully meeting the health needs of patients and overcoming the fragmented health care delivery system.

Harvey Fineberg, M.D., Ph.D, President, Institute of Medicine said, "The IOM is pleased to host this Summit at such a critical juncture in the trajectory of health care in America."

Ralph Snyderman, M.D., Chair, Summit Planning Committee, said, "As many of us are keenly aware, the current U.S. health care system is far from integrated in any sense of the word. It is reactive to disease events, fragmented, expensive, and ineffective in promoting prevention, continuity of care, and effective engagement of the patient. With the twin challenges of an economic crisis and health care that is increasingly unaffordable and often ineffective, the time for reform is now. This healthcare crisis will require innovative solutions and models of care that depart in fundamental ways from the "sick care" system we have today."

The 600 stakeholders in attendance echoed these feelings and peppered their comments with words like "we need a revolution", "we need to blow this system up and start over". Leaders in the industry such as Dean Ornish and Mehmet Oz gave testimony to Congress on the efficacy of integrative healthcare. This culmination of leading thinkers in healthcare happened over 2 years ago. Since then, no change.

Why do we need a revolution? Because change happens slowly or not at all and time is of the essence.

Self care is the innovative solution and a time tested model of care. Mothers, the Original Primary Care Physicians, have generations of evidence based outcomes. Self care is the disruptive innovator that we need to start the turn around to mindful, responsible, affordable, safe healthcare and personal responsibility for prevention and promotion of a wellness culture. This is the legacy of healthcare that is incumbent upon us to leave to our children.

It is often the women who foment revolutions. Women understand oppression, lack of freedom, lack of equality, powerlessness. Women are in the position to care for the health of their families, yet, they are shackled to one system of medicine. This prevailing system threatens to bankrupt us on many levels.

It is time to take back our power. It is time to educate yourself, invest in your healthcare. Create a culture of wellness to bask in, to flourish in.

If not now, when?

Nancy Gahles, DC, CCH, RSHom(NA)
Belle Harbor, New York
March 2012

INTRODUCTION

It is my mission, in writing this book, to share my insights, wisdom, experience, techniques and strategies as guideposts for you to use when creating your own self care plan.

By way of introduction, my name is Nancy Gahles. That is the simplest form of who I am. My work here is toiling in the field of humanity. I quite like it. It is a garden of delights.

I am an entrepreneur in the healthcare world. I operate my own healthcare business as an integrative healthcare practitioner specializing as a Doctor of Chiropractic and a Certified Classical Homeopath. I am also an Ordained Interfaith Minister. I found that the "business" of becoming well necessitated incorporating mind, body and spirit in the business plan. Thus, I pursued the path of interfaith studies in order to accommodate people of all faiths with a true understanding of their belief system. Beliefs are the result of practiced thoughts. These thoughts create our reality. Sickness, that is, the way in which we become sick, is often an out picturing of our thoughts. The way in which we find our way back to wellness, or wholeness, can be found through our belief system. Likewise, our belief system is what sustains us through the journey and what ultimately gives meaning and purpose to our lives.

I am a mother, from which I have been taught the most profound lessons of truly birthing each moment with unconditional love. I am a wife, which has humbled me to a place where I had to let go of that precious ego and actually see the Divine in another, every day, day in and day out. Sometimes it was shining brightly for all the world to see and other times, I could see but through the murky glass.

I am a freelance writer who translates these experiences into essays that make people laugh, cry and think about changing themselves and the human condition that surrounds them.

All of this wisdom has led me to formulate certain strategies for meeting the challenges that presented themselves to me while endeavoring to meet my goals and fulfill my Purpose in life whilst being in the entanglement of human relationship. No small feat but, as I always say, "To be a woman is not for the faint of heart."

While caring for people who are in pain, I understood that this is an issue for all who struggle for health. It is a challenge for all who wish to be whole and happy. The issue is the struggle for health. Once we have lost our way, the road home seems very far off. It can be daunting, but it is possible to get back to a state of well being. The challenge is to dig deep for motivation and then put your thoughts into action.

Possibilities, choice and freedom to put your choices into action as they fit into alignment with your particular purpose in life, is the right and privilege of every human being.

It is my intention in writing this book to inform, educate and empower you to become an active co-creator of your healthcare so as to meet your goals. Health, harmony and happiness. Laudable goals to be sure. This is the "stuff" of which Life is made. Our forefathers were insistent that the pursuit of life, liberty and happiness were expressly written into our Declaration of Independence precisely because they knew the value of freedom in all of its dimensions. Indeed, the prevailing thoughts of that time, the late 1700's, were echoed in the field of medicine as well. Dr. Samuel Hahnemann, the founder of a system of medicine called homeopathy, championed this system as an avenue to creating freedom from disease. In his seminal work, *Organon of the Medical Art*, 1755, he wrote about the life force in health and disease. He said, "In the healthy human state, the spirit-like life force (autocracy) that enlivens the material organism as dynamis, governs without restriction and keeps all parts of the organism in admirable, harmonious, vital operation, as regards both feelings and function, so that our indwelling, rational spirit can freely avail itself of this living, healthy instrument for the higher purpose of our existence."

My vision is a world where every person can be in charge of their own healthcare by understanding the link between what makes us tick and what makes us sick. By accessing that information and using it to create health through self care, you develop a personal responsibility that you can count on. Self reliance breeds self control in the true sense of the word. A woman of great self-reliance, Katherine Hepburn, put it aptly when she said, " As one goes through life one learns that if you don't paddle your own canoe, you don't move".

Ralph Waldo Emerson, an American Transcendentalist philosopher, wrote an essay entitled Self-Reliance, one of the central doctrines of which was "Trust thyself".

One learns to trust oneself through experience.

So, without further adieu, and to paraphrase the words of my favorite protagonist, Max, in *Where The Wild Things Are,* LET THE WILD RUMPUS BEGIN!

CHAPTER 1

THE STORY BEGINS

"It's a virus. There is nothing we can do for that." "You just have to live with it."

These words are among the most depressing words you'll hear when a loved one is sick. They instill a spirit of hopelessness and despair. How do you cope with the idea that there is nothing that can help you when you are suffering? How are you supposed to live with pain or suffering on a daily basis?

When medicine fails, what do you do?

My journey to the heart of healing began when my son was diagnosed with reactive airway disease at one-year of age. Without mincing words or making it too complicated for me, the doctor simply told me that my son had asthma.

This diagnosis was the culmination of his first year on this planet wherein his lungs appeared to be his sensitive organ. He would come down with a cold and within 24 hours he would begin coughing and have difficulty breathing. The coughing, I could deal with. It's the difficulty breathing that's a whole other matter. Generally, the cold would appear as mild nasal symptoms during the day leading me to believe he would move through it easily. Yet, more often than not, by midnight or thereafter, he would be in distress with asthmatic breathing.

There is little else more horrifying than finding yourself at home, alone, in the middle of the night with a baby, your child, who can't breathe.

When I was a little girl, we had a pediatrician who came to the house on occasions like this. Asthma ran in our family. I can remember him walking around our living room with my baby brother cradled over his arm while he patted and rubbed the congestion from his lungs. He talked and laughed with my parents and was an inestimable source of comfort.

When my son's attacks first came on so suddenly and in the middle of the night, I, likewise, called my pediatrician. The doctor on-call did get back to me and advised me to go to the emergency room. The very thought of taking my son to the emergency room sent shivers up my spine. Having put myself through chiropractic school working in the emergency room of a hospital, it was clear that I would be rendered powerless if I made that choice. The fact that I live on a peninsula with one, less than ideal, hospital made the decision easy for me. I would wait until morning and meet the doctor in the office.

The night of quiet desperation, as I now fondly recall it, was replete with steam baths, chiropractic treatment, lung taps, vaporizers, essential oils, massages and an endless petition of prayers as I watched him breathe and kept my eyes fixed on the face of the clock. Time passes slowly when you are watching every breath your child takes.

At 8:30 AM, I bundled him up and drove furiously to the doctor's office, prepared to camp out on his doorstep until 9AM. When the doors opened, his office manager showed me to an exam room and, observing the distress my son was in, called the doctor and got permission to start him on a nebulizer treatment to open his airways. About 20 minutes later, my pediatrician casually sauntered in, after biking to the office, and directed the usual care plan of antibiotics and nebulizer treatments. I was underwhelmed, yet I felt as if I was held hostage. I had no other options to choose from.

This pattern of colds turning into asthma continued from the spring until the following autumn. I began to observe the pattern. There was a cycle to his symptoms. It had happened last year and again this year when we were sitting in temple during Rosh Hoshana. I noticed that he breathed "that way." It was wheezing.

On this last occasion, I was fortunate to be sitting next to a nurse practitioner when he flared up. I asked her, "Is he wheezing?"

She looked at him, then back at me and nodded knowingly. She followed me home after the service to write a prescription for Albuterol for more nebulizer treatments. It was then that I was told that he should be placed on a program of daily inhalation treatments with a drug called Cromalyn, using a mask over his face morning and night for a year.

Once again, I was absolutely horrified! I knew, in my heart of healing hearts, that there had to be something better... curative. I had no intention of creating the mindset for him of being "an asthmatic," nor did I want him on daily medication at his young age.

It was at this point that I set out to find the elusive "something else." I knew that this system of healthcare, allopathic medicine, could not give me the solutions I needed for my son. My pediatrician could be there to provide medicine during the times of crisis, but, there were no remedies, only the theory that he might outgrow it. This left me alone to cope with the next 10 to 14 years of nighttime desperation and crisis intervention.

The fact that I was a health care professional, and an alternative one at that, was definitely in my favor. I was already mentally and emotionally prepared to look outside the box.

I was inspired to take action because there was a void in the prevailing system of healthcare. I was open to changing the paradigm that medicine holds all the answers. I was ready to change the credence that I had no power or authority to make medical decisions to care for my own child. I was ready to take that leap of faith. To believe that there was something else that could heal my son of his tendency to this type of illness. And I believed that I could take action on my own.

Although drugs are efficient in many cases, and medical technology and surgical interventions are areas of necessity, I am grateful for all the advances in this realm, and I use all the modalities that exist in healing as they are called for on a case by case basis.

I began my search by going back to the many books in my office and reading everything I could about lungs, allergies, reactive airway disease, asthma, the causes and the current treatments. That was 20 years ago. Today there is a world of knowledge at our fingertips in an instant by using the Internet. I spoke to colleagues, patients and friends, gathering information as I listened to their stories and heard the ways in which they had traversed the same path.

Stories are our way of externalizing our suffering. The ways in which people suffer from the same condition is always a source of insight for me. The diagnosis may be the same, but the manner in which the person experiences that condition is always a personal experience. For example, when my son begins to have difficulty breathing, he is very relaxed, and will work on his computer or watch television to distract himself. One of my patients becomes weepy, whining and clingy when he can't breathe. Another becomes quite agitated and fearful of dying.

I took careful note of the individual expression of the disease and continued my search for "something" that would address this individualization. I asked these questions," If the cause is a bacteria, why does the antibiotic work for some and not every case?" "Why is a person prone to this condition, and why does it repeat itself?" "Why doesn't the treatment cure the condition?"

In my experience, when one has the intention to heal and the perseverance to follow your intuition, paths open for you to follow. I was led to study about a system of medicine called homeopathy. I now gratefully call it the "missing link" in healthcare.

According to the National Institute of Health's component called the National Center for Complementary and Alternative Medicine (NCCAM), homeopathy is classified as a whole medical system. Homeopathic medicine is defined in this context ..."whole medical systems are built upon complete systems of theory and practice. Often, these systems have developed apart from and earlier than the conventional medical approach used in the United States." (http://nccam.nih.gov/health/whatiscam/#4).

I was immediately impressed by the fact that the whole person is considered when treating with homeopathic remedies. In the case of my son, the homeopath I consulted asked numerous questions about things like his food cravings, his desire for hot or cold environment, his temperament, his fears, his bowel movements, the quality of his sleep and more. He went into depth on each answer and into each organ system and behavioral peculiarity.

At the conclusion of the consultation, he prescribed a homeopathic remedy that had taken into account the whole person of my son. It is one of the laws of homeopathy called Totality of Symptoms. It made perfect sense. This is exactly what I had been searching for. The remedy that was prescribed was one that fit my son perfectly. Individualizing the remedy to the person is the keystone of specific treatment in homeopathy. Unlike allopathic medicine, every person suffering asthma will not receive the same remedy. Caution must be exercised when using self-care to be certain that you do not fall prey to asking your neighbor what they used for a certain condition and then giving that remedy to yourself or anyone else. There are rules of prescribing in homeopathy that are easy to follow. Booksellers for a list of books for beginners that contain the philosophy of homeopathy and how to use it can be found in the Resource section at the end of this book.

Following the homeopath's directions, the remedy was to be taken one time only and I was to observe his reaction and orientation toward wellness. This is another law of homeopathy called the Minimum Dose. Simply put, use the smallest dose of medicine to stimulate the organism to right itself. "Less is more" is a familiar saying that is appropriate when treating illness. Give a little and wait a lot, is a favorite adage of mine. The body has innate intelligence and will respond to a well chosen impetus to self-healing. In my opinion, this is the only true and lasting healing there is.

In my healer's heart of hearts, I knew that the "something else" that I had been looking for was homeopathy. In my mother's heart of hearts, I was immensely satisfied to have a place to start in healing my son. I was equally thrilled to have a professional that I could consult with on an ongoing basis to follow my son through and to the end of this cycle of illness.

I was encouraged by the fact that he would understand my son's predispositions and sensitivities and would be able to help me in an emergency as well as mentor me to be able to prescribe for my son in the dark, desperate hours of the night.

Information, education and teamwork in caring for my child hit just the right note. I was now singing my own song of freedom and empowerment!

THE HOMEOPATHIC REMEDY

Homeopathic remedies are classified as over the counter drugs (OTC) and are regulated by the Food and Drug Administration (FDA). They are safe and easy to use for self limiting conditions by each and every person. So, just what is a self limiting condition anyway? A self limiting condition is a term we use for the diseases that, when left alone, will run their natural course. A self limiting condition is one that usually stops or ends on its own without therapy or assistance. Earaches, cough, colds, influenzas, sore throats and many viral diseases are examples of self limiting conditions which must run their natural course in order for the body to mobilize its own immune system, mount a proper defense and repair itself. Allowing the body the time and space to perform this inherent function has the added benefit of increasing immunity to the invading virus or pathogen the next time it comes into contact with it.

Homeopathic remedies are used in self care to relieve pain and discomfort and to hasten the healing process. Reducing both severity and duration of an illness while increasing stamina is a hallmark of homeopathic treatment. Recovery is quicker and the lassitude, weakness and fatigue that often drags on for weeks after an illness is eliminated with the well selected remedy.

It certainly behooves one to learn enough about homeopathy in order to select the correct remedy even for simple conditions like coughs, colds, teething and earaches in children as well as the viral syndromes in adults.

An excellent resource is the National Center for Homeopathy (NCH). This is the world's only consumer based, open membership organization that is dedicated to homeopathy. It is open to all people interested in homeopathy from regular folk to licensed health care providers to manufacturers, writers, media representatives and political advocates. The National Center for Homeopathy raises awareness of homeopathy throughout the world. NCH protects your right to choose homeopathy as a healthcare modality and protects your access to it.

I suggest that you visit the National Center for Homeopathy's website where you will find a plethora of information about state of the art education, community, networking opportunities, study groups, conferences, social media, how to find a remedy and how to locate a practitioner and more. Go to www.nationalcenterforhomeopathy.org for information.

TRUST THYSELF

Even though I am a doctor, I have been conditioned to believe that when it comes to any symptoms not related to my specialty, chiropractic, I had better ask my medical doctor. It is a bit more than conditioned actually, it is a legal restriction. Chiropractors are thoroughly trained in diagnosis and pathology of all organ systems and sit for the same exams as medical doctors to this point and then go on to pursue specific studies in our specialty of the spine and neuro-musculo-skeletal system. As a matter of licensure, doctors of chiropractic are restricted to diagnosis and treatment of the spine only. Of course, I can auscultate the lungs and determine that there is a wheeze and then refer the patient to a medical doctor for treatment. In the case of my son, I began to notice the oddest thing. Whenever he would begin to get sick, I would listen to his lungs and while I heard a distinct wheeze, I would question myself. Was that really a wheeze? I knew it was and that it was a sign that he had a cold virus and that his body would react by vasospasm and production of mucous which would constrict his airways. I also knew that I could give him his homeopathic remedy and the symptoms would abate as his body was stimulated to heal itself. A certain sense of panic arose in me that if I was wrong, my son would suffer and perhaps die. I always felt compelled to take him to the pediatrician who would confirm my instincts and observations by telling me that it was a cold virus and that he should take an antibiotic and the nebulizer treatments every four hours and as a preventive for a few days thereafter. While we know that colds are viral in origin, it is standard of care for many pediatricians to give an antibiotic prophylactically, that is, to prevent the occurrence of a secondary infection, such as bronchitis, as a result of the cold. It has become common practice of late to routinely add a steroid to the nebulizer treatment to control inflammation. This was not a path that I felt was in the best interest of my son.

Disempowered as I felt on many occasions, I gradually began to trust myself, the gentle action of homeopathy and my son's own ability to heal himself given the right stimulus.

Gifted with the process of homeopathy, I began to understand how healing actually takes place. In fact, I learned what healing actually is. It is not merely the absence of symptoms. True healing is a manifestation of the whole person, body, mind, emotion and spirit in equilibrium. Health is the harmony of the whole person. A symphony of all the instruments in the orchestra, playing your song. In perfect pitch. Music to your ears. You feel it, you know it by the sensation it evokes in you. You are playing your signature song, your unique contribution to the song of the cosmos. This inner feeling is the one that propels you forward. It puts a spring in your step and adds a glow to your face. People who whistle while they work are mirroring the interior song of joy. People who are healthy are more productive at work. They are fully present and engaged.

As human beings, we are constantly in a state of flux, of dynamic life processes ebbing and flowing in a rhythmic, cyclic fashion. The gentle balance of remaining in the center of this exquisite choreography of life is my definition of "health."

The truth is that we are humans, and as we use the vehicle of our body to transport us through this life, we will undoubtedly encounter storms and rocky roads and traumas of all sorts as well as the inherent joys of the adventure. It is the way in which these events affect us, the way in which we perceive the issue that determines how it will be interpreted through our body, mind, emotions and spirit. How we interpret dangerous, unpleasant or overwhelming information determines where we store it. If the assault on our senses is too overwhelming to handle at that moment, we might simply put it away somewhere. Basically, we suppress that which we cannot process and rightly integrate into our being. It doesn't make sense, so we store it in a place within us that has been predetermined by our belief systems.

For instance, when my father died, I was overwhelmed. His death alone was one thing, but the fact that I had to spend over six months watching him die, gradually, was simply too much for me to bear. My favorite aunt, who was also my Godmother and a left handed, single woman role model, was dying of heart disease at the same time. It was too much sadness and too much grief for me to process at once. But, what was I to do? I had a three year old daughter and a one and a half year old son at home along with my husband and a full time chiropractic practice. I had to go on.

According to my Catholic upbringing, it is customary to mourn for three days, bury the dead and return to your normal life. I made a courageous attempt to do just that, however, my system was on overload, and I wasn't listening. The truth is, I didn't even know I was supposed to listen. I didn't even know *how* to listen. *What was I supposed to listen for?*

The week following my father's burial, I was driving to meet my mom at the nursing home where my aunt was dying. I had with me a marble urn for her to look at and decide if it would be a proper receptacle for my dad's ashes. I remember arriving at the nursing home and upon entering the room and seeing my aunt's face, I had to lie down on the bed. I felt totally dissociated from my body. I was numb with shock and grief.

I left to return home and wept the whole way. I cried and cried. As I went to reach for a tissue, I lost control of the car and hit a tree. I awoke to the bright lights of the ambulance as they cut me out while I hung upside down in my overturned car. The injuries, concussion and subsequent bouts of anxiety and depression brought me face to face with homeopathy once again.

It was during the process of my healing that I came to understand the power of grief and the need to experience it until you are able to integrate it rightly into your whole being. The homeopathic remedy I was given afforded me the opportunity to experience the subtle shift in consciousness that gradually revealed peace and a sense of harmony with the birth-death cycle. I was able to "see" that it is one continuum of the soul. Oddly enough, nearing the end, my dad once said to me, "It's the birth-death cycle, Nance. I am on this end now."

One of my patients, Sally, aptly calls this sensation "the Divine shift." It is a shift in consciousness that allows one to heal from the inside out. The way in which a homeopathic remedy addresses all the symptoms a person is expressing in body, mind, emotion and spirit causes a subtle shift in energy that one experiences almost immediately. The homeopathic remedy that is most like your state of suffering will cause a resonance to restore homeostasis or equilibrium to the whole being. I do not know of any other system of medicine that can accomplish this with the minimal dose of a safe, gentle and effective substance. I do know that allopathic medicine would have suggested anti-anxiety or anti-depressive medications that would only serve to suppress symptoms on a daily basis. Once the medication stops, the symptoms would return. Besides the fact that these medications have a host of side effects associated with them, where is the healing? Who is there to listen to the whole story of your suffering and prescribe on that totality? Who can interpret the language of your suffering and match that with a remedy that comes from nature that is perfectly similar to your suffering? This is the job of a homeopath. It is another one of the laws of homeopathy called the Law of Similars. It is also the job of the person who seeks the help of a homeopath. One has to be able to tell the story of their suffering on every level and with honesty in order to be a co-creator of their healing. It is a matter of tuning in to your Self, the Source of all. The place where creation happens.

CHAPTER 2

THE LANGUAGE OF OURSELVES

Our physical bodies speak a language through the senses. Our five senses interpret our experience of the environment in which we live and give us feedback through our central nervous system. The different organ systems speak to us in the language of sensation.

Our mental and emotional bodies speak to us through thoughts and feelings. These senses are often called extra-sensory or those senses that are outside of the five senses of taste, touch, sight, hearing and smelling. The mouth, skin, eyes, ears and nose are the organs that receive and interpret information from the external environment for your body to internalize and use for efficient functioning.

There are no specific organs of extra sensory perception. Thoughts are the product of the intellectual mind. Thoughts are our perception of an experience or event. The thoughts that we produce by mental activity constitute an idea or conception that we create based upon that experience or event. That thought becomes the "stuff" of our opinion or our point of view from that vantage point of experience.

I have always found this type of processing fascinating. There can be several people witnessing the same event and each will have their own interpretation of what happened. We see this in courtroom dramas where there are several witnesses to a crime and each of them renders a different description of the suspect and the way in which the crime happened. We "see" experiences through our own lens. Our interpretation gives rise to judgment and beliefs. The way in which we perceive is an expression of our uniqueness. Our perception colors our world and allows us to paint our own portrait of life.

This same perception creates a language of its own. The language your Self speaks is one that makes sense to you and you alone. In times of crisis, you might become so overwhelmed that you are rendered speechless, in your body and in your mind. The very thought of that crisis is banned from your consciousness. You may have heard the term spoken," Perish the thought!" This is often said in a humorous way to indicate that something is simply too terrible to be thought of. In fact, that terrible thought cannot be destroyed and so it is put somewhere in your being, stored for future reference. You are the steward of that thought and you know where the treasure is buried. Sometimes, we forget where we put it. It then becomes the homeopath's job to find the key to the safe. Like a safe cracker, we put our ear to the door and listen carefully to the tumblers until it all falls into place.

In a homeopathic consultation, I have often heard the language of those thoughts being played out through anxiety or disturbed sleep. Thoughts that are not rightly integrated are relegated to the unconscious. They are not allowed to be present in daily consciousness. "Perish the thought!"

Persistent or tormenting thoughts are the mind's way of telling you that they need to communicate something to you. Something unresolved, unfinished, not integrated.

In my case, I was in a state of grief when I had the auto accident. I simply could not get over the fact that my Dad had died and that my aunt was dying. I went back about my usual activities of life, but I was carrying an overwhelming sadness within. I lost control of my car and for me—that was the language of losing control in my life. As a doctor, I was not able to save my father. I felt guilty over that. Of course, one rationally understands that I *should not* have those thoughts, nonetheless, I did, and they were so powerful that they had to be sublimated so that I could function. My body was not deterred in its effort to bring me back into a balanced state, and so it kept up its relentless task of showing me symptoms, veritable road signs, to bring me back home.

Home seems a long way off when you have lost a loved one, especially a parent. I would cry all the time, "for no reason"; I had a severe burning rash on my throat and overwhelming panic attacks, again, "for no reason". Well, reason was not operational in my case. I remember standing in front of the refrigerator, with the door open, tapping my foot and saying, "What would make me happy?" There was not a food on earth that could fill up that void.

The rash on my throat was the symptom that got my attention. The burning, bright red rash on my throat for all the world to see was the fire that had to be put out first.

I consulted a homeopath with whom I had studied a few years previously. He took an hour or so to "take my case" as it is called in homeo-speak. He inquired about the health and function of all my body's systems and then went further into the grief, the accident, my sleep, dreams and feelings on their deepest level. The remedy that he selected for me was one that I had self medicated with at the funeral. I hadn't realized that the rash was an expression of my grief. I thought that I had cleverly suppressed it but here was an actual red flag! This was the one symptom that I was not willing to live with. That's another characteristic of individuality. The symptoms one will accept and the ones they will not. I have often found myself remarking, " But how could you live like that??" in astonishment over another person's coping style. As the saying goes, "one man's meat is another man's poison." My poison was the rash. My skin was the vehicle of expression and the rash was the language it spoke. The rash was the key to where I had buried the treasure. The treasure was my freedom from the entanglement of grief.

The homeopath was able to interpret my language. He was able to prescribe a remedy that literally unloosed my tongue. A homeopathically prepared substance, diluted and succussed to a point where it resonated similarly to my state of being, stimulated a shift in consciousness within me that sent waves of information over the internet of my cells bringing all of my systems into harmony which facilitated a return to home, that is, homeostasis, as it is called in scientific language. The remedy selected for me was Ignatia Amara, a plant remedy that covers the emotions of grief along with the physical skin symptoms that I was experiencing.

Feelings are healing, so we don't want to rid ourselves entirely of them even if they are disturbing. I learned to use my feelings as an indicator of my sensitivities and as a barometer of the intensity of my perceptions.

Marriage, children and the daily challenges of life and practice have been my greatest teachers. I am a part of a family of love that extends from my birth family, my family of choice, and to my friends and patients and beyond. This network of support has, on numerous occasions, confirmed for me the undeniable link to a web of energy that transcends our understanding of finite matter, time and space.

I now understand that when I "feel" something, I need to listen to the language, the one that I have created, and to give it the time and attention that it requires. Feelings are more ethereal than thoughts and because of this they can be relegated to the status of second class citizens in the country of your self. Feelings do not have to be given credibility. We are taught that feelings are not credible when they are not based on fact or reason. Feelings that cannot be substantiated by hard evidence are discounted. By their nature, feelings are not based on fact and should not be. Feelings are an extra sensory perception. They are a way of perceiving through a higher faculty than thinking. Feelings exist in the vital body and are represented in the material body for our analysis and conscious understanding. The way that we understand what we are feeling and how are bodies are out picturing this feeling is by focusing our attention. By becoming quiet, being present in the moment, we are available to be conscious of possibilities. As all the possibilities that exist appear in our consciousness, we are given the opportunity to choose those that are in alignment with our purpose. When our purpose is to heal ourselves, we focus our consciousness on the most appropriate choice that reflects that state that we desire. As we observe that state, the consciousness "collapses" and manifests that which we desire into material state.

These concepts are inherent to the field of quantum physics and have been studied and described since the early 1900's by eminent scientists such as Albert Einstein.

Recently, Dr. Luc Montagnier, foremost French virologist, Nobel Laureate and discoverer of the HIV virus, presented his current work on highly diluted substances and their influence on DNA. This postulates a theory for the mechanism of action of homeopathic remedies. "These would be the most significant experiments performed in the past 90 years, demanding re-evaluation of the whole conceptual framework of modern chemistry." -Andy Coghlan, *New Scientist* 12 January 2011.

Award winning science journalist Lynn McTaggart, published a book called *The Field*, in the course of attempting to find a scientific explanation for how homeopathy works. She says, "*The Field* created a picture of an interconnected universe and a scientific explanation for many of the most profound human mysteries, from alternative medicine and spiritual healing to extrasensory perception and the collective unconscious."

At present, the prevailing theories of the universe and how we interact as part of an interconnected network of systems puts homeopathy squarely in the field of quantum physics.

Candace Pert, a neuroscientist, provides in her groundbreaking work, *Molecules of Emotion*, a biomolecular basis for our emotions and explains how the chemicals inside our bodies form a dynamic network, linking mind and body. Ah! At last we are given permission to believe in our gut feelings. Scientific documentation is often necessary in a society that has been disenfranchised from their intuition and the right to believe in their own feelings and sensations. I am reminded here of the words of John F. Kennedy who said, "It is the belief that the rights of man come not from the State but from the hand of God."

Feelings and sensations are among the gateways to the soul of healing. For instance, one person with a headache might say that it feels as if there were a thousand little hammers in her head. Another will say that her headache feels as though it were bursting with heat.

I had a child as a patient who once told me that he felt as though there were dry stones rubbing together in his forehead causing a friction that could light a fire or an explosion. His dad was a firefighter who had died in the 9/11 disaster in New York City. The language of his pain was a graphic depiction of the event that he had experienced. A loss so overwhelming that the pain could not be integrated. He could not make sense of it. The way in which his body told the story of the pain was perfect. He has been given different homeopathic remedies along the course of his growth and development phases with remarkable results. The process of integrating an experience so overhwelming has been just that, a process. That is clearly what healing is all about.

When we are children, they are called milestones in development. The markers are determined by physical growth measures, for example, height, weight and head circumference as compared to other children in your range. We need to recognize and incorporate the other markers of growth.

Personal, individual experiences and their aftermath, in whatever level of being they are felt, are a part of the story, are integral to the person's health and harmony. Experiences are the substance of the recovery .

The language of the body is metaphorical. Just like homeopathy, the body speaks in similars. The information highway of the body/mind/emotion/spirit is clearly marked. The signs and symptoms appear as an allegory to the story of suffering and joy. This highway is replete with networks of paths and nodal points all of which point to the fact that we are an information processing system. Francis Schmitt coined the term, "information substances" to refer to the neuropeptides and receptors that Dr. Pert calls "... information molecules that are using a coded language to communicate via a mind-body network." She postulates a "law of information theory" that is, one that transcends time and space, placing it beyond the confining limits of matter and energy.

This being said, we can understand a bit more clearly the phenomenon of cellular memory. Experience is information. Once you have had an experience, the blueprint is there forever in your heart. It becomes a file in your experiential database. Retrieval of that information for purposes of accessing your highest potential is always within your power. One simply has to remember where they put it. Where did you store that information? I have a favorite saying, "At the end of every forget, I remember". Re-membering means putting the members back together again. Like a jigsaw puzzle. There are a thousand pieces thrown in the box but when they are all fit together, they make a picture. It makes sense. This is how one begins the healing process. Open the box, look at all the pieces and start to put them together. You can start with the border and fill in the details or you can go right to the center and work your way out to the periphery.

The way in which you carry out the process is the metaphor of your disease. Superficial disturbances first or deep seated ones. You can begin your own investigation into how you are processing and storing your information by going within. Pretend that it is your own website. Go to your home page. Home is where your story begins. You know intuitively and instinctively where home is. You also know when you are far from home and lost. Remember the stories of Lassie or other heroic animals who would walk for hundreds of miles to get back home? If they can do it, you can do it!

Now you know how to get there. Follow the trail of significant events, traumas and lifestyle changes. This reminds me of the children's story of *Hansel and Gretel* where they dropped breadcrumbs along the path into the forest so that they could find the way back home. Reality can feel like fiction when the birds eat the breadcrumbs and we can't find the markers to lead us out of the forest. It is then that we look inward to our inner compass for the route.

Never has this strategy for healing been more apropos than now. There has arisen on the health scene a new spectrum of dysfunctions that present themselves with unknown etiology (causation), and varied symptoms on the mental/emotional plane that manifest as inability to learn, communicate and socialize. How does medicine address these cases that have no germ to kill, nothing to cut out, freeze or burn off, or parts to replace? Once again, we are set adrift in the unknown territory of fear and desperation. Alone. Responsible to figure it out on your own. Or, to simply live with it.

Standing at the periphery of this dark and daunting forest, I took my daughter's hand and walked right in. I was scared and I was confident. I was scared because I was unprepared for all the challenges I would encounter and I was confident that all the answers would appear if I simply kept putting one foot in front of the other and tuned in with all my senses for the signs along the way. Unfortunately, there were no breadcrumbs to follow so I paced myself to the rhythm of my heart. There is no sharper explorer or relentless warrior than the heart of a mother searching for healing for her child.

My first born, my daughter, began life as the delight of our lives. I took her everywhere with me. I bundled her into a backpack every morning and drove into my office in Manhattan where she had a place in my consultation room. She was exposed to all manner of situations and people and was bright, alert, sociable and smart. Being an avid reader myself, she was read to constantly from every genre of literature. Twenty years ago, baby sign language was not in vogue, but if it was, I probably would have taught her that. We danced, sang and frequented concerts for babies and later the Young People's Symphony series at Lincoln Center.

Gifted programs were in vogue at the time and so at the age of three and a half, she was "tested" for acceptance into a gifted Pre-K program at a progressive public school. I remember distinctly the day I brought her to the psychologist's office for the battery of psychological and social testing required to determine her budding genius status or lack thereof.

The woman psychologist came out, took Jade's hand and led her willingly away to another room. I sat on pins and needles waiting...anticipating. After about an hour, I heard the tapping footsteps of her little red patent leather shoes coming down the hall, alone. I asked her what happened and she replied, quite matter-of-factly, "She wasn't nice to me, so I wasn't nice to her." I, quite naturally, was horrified. A few minutes later, the psychologist emerged from her room and told me, in a brusque manner, that at one point in the testing, Jade stopped being the testee and became the tester directing the psychologist to accomplish the tasks requested of her. I was a bit surprised at how flummoxed she was at Jade's behavior. After all, she *is* a professional in this field. Her abrupt "The testing is over" statement assured me that she was not kidding. Forlorn, I went home, kissing goodbye to the genius program. It so happened, however, that her scores were "very superior" and, as noted in the letter of recommendation, would have been higher had she continued testing.

Off to genius school she went and continued uneventfully until the end of first grade when, at the closing theatrical performance, it became patently obvious that all the other children were reading their lines and Jade was having them read into her ear and repeating them back. She couldn't read.

I knew she was struggling with whole sentences, however her teacher had assured me that she was fine and that every child "gets it" in their own time. At some point, she told me, the light just goes on. Not willing to sit in total darkness waiting for that inevitable spark of light, I employed a tutor for the summer. This was to be the first in a long line of tutors throughout her life in my constant quest for "something else" than the public school education, a system that was failing her. "Something else" that would spark that light. She couldn't read and so they pulled her out of class to give her extra reading. More of what she couldn't do only spiraled her into an attitude of failure and incompetence.

Not being able to read was not a disease or was it? I consulted the full spectrum of medical specialists from eye doctors to neurologists to learning specialists and beyond. She was not dyslexic; eyes were fine, no neurological issues. There was nothing wrong with her. Enter the frustrated heart of a mother. What do we do when medicine has no answer? What do you do when you instinctively know that something is amiss but it falls below the category of a diagnosable condition that can be treated by the prevailing medical model?

I did the things that were available to me. I took the well traveled path. The known and acceptable route. I had her put into the class with a teacher of phenomenal reputation. I had her tutored. I spent endless hours reading to her and helping with her assignments. She was normal in every way and a happy, social child. The day I walked her to her second grade classroom and saw the stack of textbooks on her desk I knew we were in trouble. Sure enough, by the second week of school, as they were lining up to enter the building, the teacher looked up over her head and mouthed the words, "She is really struggling". Not exactly music to my ears. I felt my stomach drop into my shoes, and I slogged home in them weary from the weight.

What to do when there are no answers in the mainstream forums? My intention was to do everything I could to make certain that her self esteem did not suffer while I figured out this dilemma. This teacher accomplished that. Due to her amazing abilities, she made Jade feel confident and bright throughout the year despite her learning issues. My daughter still remembers this and loves her for it. That, by the way, is the hallmark of a true teacher.

At the end of third grade, in our public school system, one is required to take a series of standardized tests in Math and English. I now refer to them by their rightful name, bastardized tests. The amount of preparation required for these tests has been responsible for the elimination of study in the sciences and history classes, among others, the impact of which is educationally devastating. The emphasis that is put on performance for these tests has wreaked havoc on the children emotionally. My daughter was one such casualty.

I remember when she walked into my office at the end of third grade after they had announced the scores. She had performed poorly. Her posture spoke the whole story. Hunched over and tapping that little foot, my eight year old announced,

"Mom, I think I am stupid." She had the look of a beautiful flower wilting. Not only did my stomach drop but my entire interior plummeted to the floor. As though listening through a tunnel, in my numbness, I heard her muffled voice attempting to explain to me, and herself, how she thought she was smart and now this test was telling her something different. It was telling her that she was, indeed, different and that difference wasn't good. Her scores clearly indicated to her that she was stupid.

I jumped into battle, waging war on this unfair system of assessing my daughter's worth and ravaging her self esteem. I stood up, looked her straight in the eye and I told her that this system of education was only one way of learning and that there are many other ways to be educated. This way was not for her. It didn't fit her unique style of learning. I surely was not going to let her fall through the cracks. Secretly, I asked myself, what did suit her best?

I took her hand and walked with her, dragged her and often carried her through the process of discovering her learning style. I donned my superhuman mother's cape and armed with not much more than moxie, I entered the dense forest of homeschooling. Lions and tigers and bears, Oh,My!

What is reading? How can you not simply learn to read? It was a conundrum for me. This was uncharted territory. I had to rely on my inner compass to show the way. I tuned in to my feelings. I listened to my intuition, I observed my daughter with an unprejudiced eye, I researched, read, consulted and assembled a team of professionals to work with.

Integrative medicine is a new concept in the healthcare system. In the case where there is no specific pathology to treat, I found that it is to your best advantage to look outside the box for something and someone else to help meet your goal to return to health and well being.

My daughter is a multi-sensory learner. This type of learning by using all of your senses along with movement is also called kinesthetic learning. We incorporate the higher levels of consciousness including intuition and social interactions via relationships as well. Let's call it "supersensory learning."

I taught my daughter how to read, firstly by exciting her about the adventure of life. Stimulating in her the desire to explore those things that she was curious about, naturally involved reading about them. Reading was always downplayed in favor of real life experience as the thought of having to read evoked anxiety and resistance. It had been tainted forever with the word "stupid."

The way in which this overwhelming thought of being stupid was displayed in my daughter was in the language she used to express it. She was not able to read a sentence to completion and understand what she read. She had difficulty sounding out the words. The words jumped off the page as she tried to follow them. She would put her head down and fall asleep. Procrastination was her watchword. It was this language that a homeopath used to prescribe a remedy for her that helped tremendously in reducing the anxiety associated with reading and enhancing her stamina to stay focused on a page.

There are instances when more than one therapeutic modality can and should be used simultaneously. In this case, the subtleties of balancing the sympathetic and parasympathetic activity of the central nervous system was important to the development of her ability to process information as she read it. Discoveries in the world of neuroanatomy as to what parts of the brain are involved in processing information enabled me to treat her with cranial therapy yielding remarkable results. To this, I added specific chiropractic manipulations that addressed areas of chronic subluxation, or misalignments of the vertebra, that created an interference with her optimal neurologic functioning. The issue of low motor tone, as it related to her neck flexor muscles, was also considered with regard to weakness of the occipital-ocular reflex required for facility in reading. I noticed that after her strengthening exercises and yoga poses she was able to hold her head up longer without muscle fatigue and was able to read through sentences for a longer period of time. I likewise noted my guilt at recalling how I had let her stand or carried her rather than insist that she lie on her belly and crawl. She never liked that position as a baby and I never made her stay in an uncomfortable position. Well, that was my first child and who knew? At this point we revisited the cross crawl patterning that is essential for proper brain development and creation of a strong curve in the cervical spine.

Lifestyle choices that allow you to choose the environment for learning is another avenue to follow. At the end of one year of homeschooling, I selected a private school for her. This school provided a safe, homey feeling. The class size was small so that she could have the individual attention she needed. The emphasis in their teaching was on the celebration of each person's uniqueness and their contribution to the group learning was empowering. There was never any competition and, halleluiah, no standardized testing. My little flower flourished here and grew into a beautiful, self confident person. I can't say that she loves to read, but I will say that in her first year of college she came into my room, book in hand and announced, "Mom, I am going to read a book." My mother heart of hearts thumped with joy. Eighteen years later! The light was on! I could die a happy woman. I used to teasingly tell her that I wanted this epitaph on my tombstone, *SHE DIED TRYING TO GET HER DAUGHTER TO READ*.

Coordinating the types of treatments that were best for her required diligent observation and lots of trials and errors. The truth of health care is that it is largely "self care." One must be ready and responsible to embark on the journey with the understanding that you are forging a new path for yourself. You are the only one who can develop the information about what makes you tick and what makes you sick. All else is commentary, as the wisdom traditions say. Once you have a good understanding about your own process, then you can assemble a team of practitioners to support you.

I envision a world where you are able to use your self knowledge to create a team of professionals with whom you consult on health issues that require a higher or different level of problem solving than you are prepared for at the time the challenge arises. The challenge arises when you become sick or dysfunctional in some way and realize that you need professional help.

In our culture, we are taught to seek medical attention when we are sick. Classic interventions are drugs or surgery. These are what I call "last ditch efforts or, "heroic measures". By the time that you are in this state, reason may not prevail. It is very difficult to think clearly and calmly when you are sick. In fact, that is a predominant feature of disease. Judgment calls that are made from weakness and fear do not usually bode well for short or long term tresolution. When in this state, we feel helpless and generally cede power to a decision maker other than ourselves for the care we need. Crisis intervention is NOT healthcare. Treating acute sickness is NOT healthcare in its true form. These are emergencies and there is a place for them to be addressed in our prevailing system of medicine. There are all too many disorders that are so called "functional" for which allopathic medicine has no answer.

Interestingly, the issue that my daughter recovered from, is now termed a "visual processing disorder." There are processing disorders related to hearing as well called "auditory processing disorders." Asperger's Syndrome is a situation where social cues are not interpreted or processed properly. Errors in the way in which we process information have now been recognized in the healthcare arena as an issue. The ubiquitous question remains. *What to do for it?* The identification of the individual characteristics of each person's experience is the key to the buried treasure. The discovery of the treasure is part of the fun of life. Life's exuberance is revealed in how we traverse the unchartered territory. Treasure hunts have always been a great source of delight at children's parties. Why? Because there are the elements of thrill, adventure, discovery, challenge, failures, obstacles and twists and turns in the course of events. It makes us laugh along the way. I once read that children laugh an average of 146 times a day. Adults laugh an average of 4 times a day. That, my friends, is not healthy.

The treasure hunt engages our ability to persist in the face of adversity and it builds character strengths. Adversity, yes, a bit of suffering, shows us what we are made of. We need to overcome the belief that we have to immediately get rid of any pain we have, within reason of course. In most instances, we need to be with the suffering long enough to discover the source so that we can correct it. When we are enabled, through the indiscriminate use of drugs, to suppress the symptoms, we disable the system from effectively processing information and the system shuts down. You have got to be in it to win it!

A favorite quote of mine by Annie Besant in her book, *Wisdom*, aptly describes courage by saying, "Never forget that Life can only be nobly inspired and rightly lived if you take it bravely and gallantly, as a splendid adventure in which you are setting out into an unknown country, to face many a danger, to meet many a joy, to find many a comrade, to win and lose many a battle."

The force that drives us to persist in the face of failure and defeat is an intrinsic one that has been likened to the quest for the Holy Grail, the ineffable that is earnestly desired. It is the pursuit of our highest potential. It is our innermost desire to connect with and unleash all the abundance of the Universe and have it manifest through us in the intentions, thoughts and actions of our daily Life. This is what I know as health.

Dr. Samuel Hahnemann, the founder of homeopathy, in his seminal work, *Organon of the Medical Art*, describes health in this way: "In the healthy human state, the spirit-like life force (autocracy) that enlivens the material organism as dynamis, governs without restriction and keeps all parts of the organism in admirable, harmonious, vital operation, as regards both feelings and functions, so that our indwelling, rational spirit can freely avail itself of this living, healthy instrument for the higher purposes of our existence."

The quest for the treasure, the Holy Grail, is simply, a return to our true selves, a return home. As Dorothy discovered, in *The Wizard of Oz*, after a long and frightful journey to find the answer from outside of herself, from the wizard, that he was merely a man behind the curtain. He could do nothing to help her. So, she hooked up with Glenda, the good witch, declared her intention to go home, clicked her heels three times in those ruby slippers and chanted, "There's no place like home!"

CHAPTER 3

GOING HOME

My mom used to read us a book by Dr. Seuss called, *Oh, The Places You'll Go*. My mom put the "fun" in dysfunctional. We laughed a lot in my family of nine and we learned to take the journey rightly. Laugh, cry and hang onto to each other for dear life!

There are many avenues into the depths of your innermost being, the place where your wisdom resides. You will discover your right path as you go. I will show you some examples of ways that I have used with success. Let us start our quest with the opening words from Dr Seuss.

> *"Congratulations!*
> *Today is your day.*
> *You're off to Great Places!*
> *You're off and away!*
>
> *You have brains in your head.*
> *You have feet in your shoes.*
> *You can steer yourself*
> *Any direction you choose.*
>
> *You're on your own. And you know what you know.*
> *And YOU are the guy who'll decide where to go."*

CHOICE

Choice. It's all about choice. And choice is freedom.

Each example of avenues to explore emphasizes a particular style of processing or learning.

Auditory means that you prefer to hear things as you more easily understand in this way.

Visual means that you learn best by reading the words or seeing a picture.

Kinesthetic means that you learn by using all of your senses together and incorporating movement.

Feel free to create your own healing path.

BREATH

The first step always begins with the breath.

Logically, we know this. Breath is the first action that indicates viable life outside the womb. It is the function that supports our every moment in life. It is the last thing we let go of as we transition from this life. In reality, we don't breathe very well, very completely or very often. Breath holding and aberrant patterns in breathing are created in response to stressors and traumas in life and become deeply ingrained in us. In my hands-on healing practice of chiropractic and craniosacral therapy, the very first thing we do is learn to breathe. The way "in" is through the breath. All wisdom traditions teach this. The breath is considered to contain all the components necessary to feed and nourish the entire being. It has been referred to as prana, chi, Holy Breath and the Holy Spirit. The breath is the portal of entry to life. The breath connects us to our Source. Heart centered breathing connects you to that place within that already "knows" – that sits in the stillness waiting to receive you. As such, it is a fine place to begin! (see video tutorial on breathing at www.drnancygahles.com)

CREATE SPACE

Create a space that feels comfortable and nurturing to you. Make it a place that you go to in order to leave your known surroundings behind. It is your sacred space. Have an area within it that you can lie down on, such as a yoga mat or blanket. Have a low seat with a back on it to support yourself during long sessions. I like the option of a meditation cushion and mat as well for shorter sitting periods. Keep it simple. The less visual distractions, the more you can focus on your thoughts, feelings and sensations. I often use a candle to begin my focusing sessions, especially when I find myself all jumbled up in the entanglements of life. Simply gazing at the flame while beginning to breathe draws you into a peaceful center. In my space I also have paper and pen for journaling. I have found that when I jot down feelings and thoughts and revelations I know I don't have to remember them as they are occurring and this allows me the freedom to keep receiving uninterruptedly. Later, as I read from my sessions, a pattern usually emerges which makes eminent sense in the whole scheme of things.

I keep a small bowl of water with which I symbolically cleanse myself before I enter into meditation. I dip my finger in the bowl and touch my brow for insight, my eyes to see clearly, my ears to hear objectively, my lips to speak my truth and my heart to receive with unconditional love.

Sound is a vibration that induces relaxation so music as well as chanting is a wonderful way to begin your inward journey. Baroque music has been said to mimic the rhythm of your heartbeat and the effects of Mozart's music has been well documented to stimulate brain waves to enhance learning and focus. I keep a collection of these works in my space and use them as I feel called to.

As I begin my breathing, I often spontaneously start to chant the word, OM. For me, the vibration of this sound is a centering experience. I feel the sensation of vibration in my body and am able to recognize this as a pattern of energy that I will meet as I go further inward on my journey. I have identified what a vibration of harmony feels like to me. I have witnessed where the vibration resonates in my body. And, more importantly, where it does not. The places that do not resonate with this frequency are the parts that are not included in the harmonious function of the whole system. These are your areas of interest. Make a note to inquire within.

After the vibration of the chant ceases, I am aware only of the rhythms and cycles of my breath. I observe the *quality* of my breath. The *depth* and *breadth* of the inspiration and the exhalation. Make a note to investigate this as it relates to the areas of non-resonance. I stay in this awareness. I observe my heartbeat. I feel the sensation, its own vibration within the chest cavity. I am aware of the way in which the heartbeat feels in connection to my breathing. I am present to the dance of life between these two exquisitely timed partners. Tango? Fox trot? Rumba? Cha-cha? This is your dance…the one that maintains your existence. Make a note of how that feels for you.

There are many ways to connect and go within that do not require sitting and chanting. The same physical, mental and spiritual effects can be had from walking in nature, swimming in the ocean, biking through trails. It is all about quieting the outer mind, connecting to the breath and being present in the moment to listen, observe, feel and intuit. The same principles apply. Be flexible and adapt these suggestions to your own style. It doesn't matter how you get there, what matters is that where you arrive is home. The place where you feel safe to explore the deepest parts of your Source energy. Your true self. For video tutorials on some of these practices go to my website www.drnancygahles.com.

I once sat in a hollowed out giant Sequoia tree in the Muir Woods in Sausalito, California where I had one of the most inexplicable spiritual experiences in my life. Being a part of the this amazing spectacle of nature was awe inspiring in a way that dwarfed my physical body and humbled me in the presence of the grandeur of this tree.

The lore of the Sequoia is that the tree is so tall that it acts as a lightening rod to catch on fire and burn off the lower branches and dead wood from the forest floor brush as a means of natural deforestation. This fire kick-starts regeneration of the seedlings which grow from the ash. The tree provides its own method of destruction and re-birth in an exquisitely orchestrated phenomenon that is thousands of years old.

I happened to be traveling at this time as a respite from a devastating business fiasco that left me bankrupt and in ruins. Sitting in the trunk of the giant Sequoia and hearing the legend of this species, illuminated my understanding of the process of natural destruction in order to clear the path for new life to grow. And it was from the seeds of this devastation that I flourished. I likened myself to the sacred mythical bird, the Phoenix, known as the firebird. The Phoenix has a 500-1,000 year life-cycle, near the end of which it builds itself a nest of twigs that then ignites, burning fiercely until both the nest and the bird are reduced to ashes. From the ashes a Phoenix egg arises, reborn anew, to live again. This symbolism, derived from my experience with nature, resonated deeply with my Source, and was the inspiration that gave me the courage to move forward and rebuild my life again. Just as the Sequoia and the Phoenix have done for thousands of years before me. I was able to believe that I could do it from the analogy with nature that I felt as I immersed myself in it. This is self care in it's fundamental glory. Experiencing deep healing by connecting to nature, to a power greater than yourself, and, *feeling* that change. *Becoming, owning* the change. Creating an experiential database in this way adds to your permanant library within.

Wayne Dyer, in his book, *Change Your Thoughts, Change Your Life*, tells us that "the reason it's crucial to have a sense of awe is because it helps loosen the ego's hold on your thinking. You can then *know* that there's something great and enduring that animates all of existence. Being in awe of that something staves off disasters because you have no fear of worldly conditions. You've kept grounded in the other-worldy power that manifests a trillion miracles a second, all of which are oblivious to your ego."

Dr. Dyer continues by saying, " I love the metaphor of nature as a guide to sage like acceptance". He references the master

Lao-tzu, who, throughout the 81 verses of the Tao Te Ching, emphasizes being in harmony with the natural world, telling you that's where you connect with the Tao.

In fact, all major religions emphasize the same principles of nature and it's ability to provoke a sense of awe, a sense of the miraculous.

The sensation of being a part of something greater than ourselves is ultimately healing in it's own right. The Bible quotes John, the apostle, in 15:4-5, "stay joined to me and I will stay joined to you. Just as a branch cannot produce fruit unless it stays joined to the vine, you cannot produce fruit unless you stay joined to me. I am the vine, and you are the branches."

Indeed, changing our thoughts about the way we perceive our "condition", is a viable way to change our health. It makes perfect sense. But, is it *common* sense?

It isn't the generally accepted way of addressing health concerns but it is the *way*, or the Tao, of nature. We *are* an integral unit of nature.

Again, Wayne Dyer puts this concept into understandable terms. "Learn about the Tao by being in perfect harmony with the environment. Think of the trees, which endure rain, snow, cold, and wind-and when the harsh times arrive, they wait with the forbearance of being true to their inner selves. As Deng Ming-Dao writes in *365 Tao :Daily Meditations:* "They stand, and they wait, the power of their growth apparently dormant. But inside, a burgeoning is building imperceptibly...neither bad fortune nor good fortune will alter what they are. We should be the same way."

Well, of course we should! How could we have forgotten this truth when nature speaks this language all around us, at every moment?

How have we become so disconnected?

As a society, we have become more industrialized, more dependent on external factors to provide us with our sustenance. We no longer believe in the sustainability of a higher consciousness. We do not believe that there is a greater power within than without.

The concept of a dual nature of the universe is a myth. In my understanding, the creation of disease comes from the belief in the duality of the universe.

Healing yourself by understanding that there is no duality is a function of higher consciousness. I believe that we are ready to take that leap of faith, believe in ourselves and use our own inner gifts to heal ourselves.

John Randolph Price, a metaphysical thinker and prolific writer on this subject, explains this concept in his own words:

"The dual nature of the universe does not exist in the True World. There is neither health nor sickness, abundance nor scarcity, peace nor conflict. God IS, the only Power, infinite and omnipresent Spirit. All else is Maya, illusory appearance projected by mind, whether judged good or bad by the seer. In Spirit, nothing is lacking, nothing is absent. Whatever is not of God does not exist. There is nothing opposed to God. Truth has no opposite; therefore, all is perfect. Spiritual consciousness knows this and does not experience duality."

Now, before you fling the book away at the mention of the word God, let me explain my use of this highly charged word. When we begin to dwell in the realms of intuition, insight and attempt to make good use of the powers of our higher consciousness, an element of the spirit enters. The awe, that ineffable something that nature bespeaks.

Poets, storytellers, philosophers, theologians over the centuries have equated this with the word God. Unfortunately, this same word has been tainted by the restrictive, exclusive, heirarchical, patriarchal and often, abusive practices of organized religion.

That said, I cite a lovely explanation of the word God by an Aramaic scholar, Dr. Neil Douglas-Klotz, from his study guide on *Original Prayer.*

"Our English word "God" is based on Germanic roots that are related to the word and concept "good"... The old Hebrew words *Elohim* or *Eloha* and the old Canaanite *Elat* as well as the Arabic *Allah* all point towards the unity of existence, embodied in a name that idealizes the sacred...According to the word

Jesus used, "God" means that no one and nothing is excluded; everything is included in Cosmic Unity".

So, let us proceed.

ACCESSING HIGHER CONSCIOUSNESS THROUGH VISUALIZATION

Imagination is a way of dwelling in another consciousness. Imagination is innate to human beings. Imagery is a Divine language, a 3-D substance that gives us knowledge about ourselves. As children, we call it day-dreaming. In present day society, this activity is frowned upon in favor of the pursuit of, what I call "artificial intelligence". That is, the didactic learning of the all important three R's. Reading, 'Riting, and 'Rithmatic. A learned mechanism of externalizing our intelligence and devaluing our inner intelligence.

Developing a practice whereby one can access higher consciousness will serve to reinforce the existence of your innate strength, confidence and the Truth of who you are.

From this place, you retrieve your wellness tools.

Creating a picture or an image in your mind's eye is a practical and easy way to guide yourself to a still place within. Guided imagery is one of the most potent tools in our toolbox for stress and pain management . Symbols connect us with archetypal memory which brings us to a place of Oneness, a place of peace. I call this place Home.

HOME

Home is where your heart is. Here you are. Home at last. Come right in. Open the door to your heart. The heart is the repository of unconditional love. Welcome!

There are four chambers. Two on the first floor and two on the second floor. You can set them up in any way that pleases you. I picture the heart as an open faced dollhouse.

The lower chambers have wing chairs and a huge fireplace in the center that spans all four chambers. This is the place where I receive guidance. It is actually a reception area of sorts. All manner of luminaries have passed through this chamber. At any given time, these hallowed halls have been graced with the presence of ascended spiritual masters, universal intelligentsia, life coaches, math tutors from another dimension, and, my Dad.

The upper chambers are for BE-ing. I go there to be. Not in the presence of any one person or thought but simply in the Presence of One. It is here where I synch up, so to speak. In my waking life, I add a file to my music library and then synch it to my iPod so I can listen to it wherever I am. That is what I do in my upper chambers. I synch to Universal Consciousness, the One Mind or All That Is. I am in the network. I feel connected. I feel whole, complete, joyous, happy, healthy and wise.

Whatever the moniker you use, the vibration is the one that you will recognize as the one that resonates in this way for you. It is like falling in love. You simply know it in every cell of your being and you want to shout it from the rooftops!

Once you know where home is, and what home feels like, you will have an unerring blueprint for it. You will have an innate guidance system that will always direct you back. The key is not to stray too far from your path. Your path will take you to fulfill your purpose in life. Just like the Yellow Brick Road. I found a delightful metaphor for this as I was driving my son to Massachusetts to look at colleges. We bought a GPS system, and I was so relieved to have someone there to tell me if I got lost. She really does know where you want to go and when you make a wrong turn she redirects you. During the drive, I made a conscious choice to deviate from the route and she sternly alerted me to "return to the highlighted route." The route on the display was clearly highlighted in yellow. The veritable Yellow Brick Road!

The analogy is that when we know where we are going and we input our destination, "she" will keep us on our path to ensure that we reach our goal. "She" is our intuition, our inner knowing, our own global positioning system. Our goal is that which is the purpose of our existence. It is that intangible state that we now know as health which is the out picturing of our vital energy manifesting as the unique individual you. The very picture of health! As a healthy, happy, whole individual you are now free to create life experiences that match this vibration. You manifest the work you do in this world, the relationships that you have and the abundance of materials that support your dream. All of these gifts allow you to be of service to your fellow humans as only you can do. Your contribution to the whole of life is only met through your service. No one else ever can, ever did, or ever will sound this note in the Grand Symphony.

What happens when, despite our best intentions, we fall off the track, become sick and can't receive the homing signals? This is the time to go into your space, take an objective look around the interior of body, mind, feelings and sensations and take stock of what is happening.

Below is a technique that I use to uncover the hidden treasure and to provide the keys for your homeopath to work with. I call it going to the Source.

GOING TO THE SOURCE

Lie comfortably and begin your breathing. Allow the breath to seek its natural rhythm. Often, when we are unwell, the breath has a different rhythm than the one which we recognize when we are at peace. Make a note of the characteristic of this breath. Is it fast? Slow? Jumpy? Is it difficult to take in the breath? Difficult to let go? What thoughts are associated with this type of breath? What feelings are associated with that thought? Where do you feel that in your body? What organ or system is representing that feeling for you?

As you begin to receive the insight, make notes. I find it useful to make a body map. Simply draw an outline of your body and fill in parts and organs where you think they ought to be. Even more interesting, draw them in where they *feel* to you.

After your session, mark the organs that were involved and the physical symptoms and thoughts, feelings and sensations associated with each. (see video tutorial at www.drnancygahles.com)

As you progress with this exercise, each day you will find patterns that emerge. You will become aware of how your feelings are speaking to you and the language that is being used to express it. Be patient with yourself. Be loving and compassionate with yourself. Allow whatever it is that comes up to be there. Being non-judgmental is key.

One of my patients recently told me that she was no longer having horrible pain in her side. She had been told she had irritable bowel syndrome but the medication wasn't helping. After taking a homeopathic remedy, she reported her ability to notice that her pain began during conversations when she got very passionate about voicing her opinion. She had come from a strong Italian background where she was hushed up and not allowed to voice her opinions. Each time she got the pain, she noticed that this was the situation. She told me that, on reflection, her passion was her pain. Her frustration and anger at being silenced fed the condition. It was only then when she realized that she was able to control the situation by choosing people to be in her life that supported her and appreciated her opinions.

Healing is a gradual process of one revelation after another. It is a joyous thing when we become aware of the fact that it is all in our control. In Napoleon Hill's book, *Think and Grow Rich,* he tells us that the only thing that makes us different from animals is that we can control our thoughts.

Fear, desperation and hopelessness derive from a sense that we have no control and all effort is fruitless. This is the "stuff" of chronic disease and disability. If, as Mr. Hill suggests, we can control our thoughts, then, after identifying them, we can change them to suit our purpose. This is the "stuff" of responsible self care and the creation of a healthy you.

CHAPTER 4

THE BUSINESS OF BEING YOU

Creating a healthy you involves the same process as creating a healthy company.

It is a complicated and heady experience, this business of being you. First of all, there is no clearly defined job description. Secondly, if you did manage to figure one out for yourself, it has the nasty propensity to keep changing just when you think you had it down pat.

It seems that just when you think you can start to coast a bit, change happens. All in a dither, you begin again to sort out the chaos, troubleshooting once again until the innate problem solver emerges and the crisis passes.

And so life goes until it becomes a wearying experience. This can be frustrating and depressing, for some, as the same old trials and tribulations arise over and over again. This is a red flag for sure that the business of being you is not yielding the returns you had anticipated.

The given is that you ARE you and that cannot be changed. You can rail at all the external factors that have caused you the grief that you are suffering with, and that may palliate your feelings for a while. The fact is that unless and until you take charge of your own business, you will never be free to be all that you can be. You will never be free from pain and suffering until you re-member your assets and re-allocate them.

Creating a business plan for yourself can be as simple as outlining the top three goals, ideas, plans or visions for your life that you would like to achieve. *If* you *knew* that you could attain these conditions in life, what would that look like for you?

What are the factors that are holding you back? Where does your resistance lie? In what tissues are your issues?

Begin to find solutions to these questions by taking time. Imagine that you are at work and a situation has come up that needs to be addressed. You must make time to sort it out.

Create a time of day where you can be in a quiet space for 20 minutes. Arrange an area for you to be in comfort. Surround yourself with objects or pictures that make you happy. Pictures of relatives or friends who supported you and loved you unconditionally are wise choices. These can be your virtual Board of Directors. Add on to the Board people, alive or dead, whom you perceive to be inspirational, motivational figures.

Awards, trophies or certificates of achievement that reflect times where you excelled in a particular endeavor are wonderful reflective pieces. When in a quandary as to how to proceed, go back to strategies that were successful for you and re-work them to suit the situation at hand. You can also recall wise elders or inspirational people and ask yourself how they would have handled such a matter.

Select a candle to focus on and a particular scent that evokes feelings of serenity. A small bowl of water that can be used to cleanse and bless yourself should be placed in front of you. You may begin by dipping your fingers in the bowl as an act of purification. You can dip your fingers in the bowl and touch your eyes, ears and lips in blessing what you see, hear and speak.

The business of being you begins when you set the stage and show up for the performance. There is a term in the business world called "presenteeism." This is used to refer to employees who show up for the job but are not fully functioning because they are ill or suffering. The quality of their work is poor and costly to their employer. You, as CEO of your own company, want to be certain to be clear and present and fully functional each day.

Getting down to business is as easy as taking your place and inhaling your first breath. Just like being born. The first breath affirms the reality of embodied consent. Your job description can come to fruition by reflecting on statements like this:

- I am me and I am part of this world by my own design and consent.
- I am the boss of myself. I create the business of my life by choosing those ideas that use my talents most effectively for my own good and the good of all.
- I choose products and services that fulfill my potential and a need in this world.
- I show up for my business every day filled with the excitement of possibilities to express myself.
- I attract like minded individuals into my business and create sustainable networks.
- The business of being me includes creating a healthy environment in my body, emotions and spirit.
- I am me and I create the most profitable business in my time simply by being a healthy, harmonious me.

As the tides of time and fortune shift, your business will be able to sustain losses when you are invested in yourself and fully diversified. Diversification is born of an inner knowing of who you are, where your susceptibilities and your strengths lie. Invest for the short term in your most susceptible areas and keep your powder dry for the long haul with regard to your strengths.

Each and every day, take your seat at the head of the boardroom table and, as CEO of yourself, go over your balance sheet and make an assessment of you. What needs to be changed, what can stay the same, what do you have to let go of and who has to be fired?

The business of being you should be the greatest adventure you will ever take. As with all businesses, it requires care and attention to details. The boss can't be away from the business for long periods of time for when the cat is away, the mice will play and you may return to a shell of a business. Bankruptcy of body, mind, emotions and spirit only occurs when you haven't shown up for work.

The business of being you is created each and every day when you take those 20 minutes and check in. That is what showing up for work means. That is when the fun begins. Creating your world of effects from your own deliberate intention is one of the most natural joys I have ever experienced. And that, my friends, is the ultimate success in the business of being a healthy, harmonious you!

INVESTMENT STRATEGIES FOR HEALTH AND PRODUCTIVITY

Now that you have a good idea of who you are, where you are going and what your strengths and weaknesses are, you are ready to develop an investment strategy in your health for present productivity and long term return on investment.

Recently, we have been shown a remarkable lesson in economics. The stock market had fallen to one of the lowest points in its history. Banks were failing and the government was called in to bail them out. The culprit? Greed. The seduction of profits in the instrument of money, bonuses and big cash payouts in severance put formerly reputable companies out of business. The CEO's were not trustworthy. We can take a lesson from history as we form our own companies and put ourselves as the CEOs. Generally, that implies that we have our own best interest at heart and will serve to increase our profit without putting the system at risk.

For our purposes, the system is the vehicle of our body and our goal is to have it serve us profitably as we maneuver our way through life to achieve our highest ideals.

Short term investments in our physical body will yield immediate returns in the form of daily energy, stamina and endurance.

Long term investments in our mental, emotional and spiritual bodies will yield returns over time in the form of happiness, nurturing relationships, security and a peacefulness that will sustain us in our "last semester of Life," as my Dad called it.

CREATING A HEALTH & HARMONY PORTFOLIO

A portfolio is a term used in finances to describe a purposeful collection of investments that reflect your lifestyle goals and risk-limiting strategy.

When creating an investment portfolio for your health, the same principles apply. There are short term investments and long term investments.

Health is your short term investment and Harmony is your long term investment. Health, in this case, is your daily level of energy and absence of disease that allows you to live your life unencumbered by physical, psychological or emotions burdens. Harmony is your quality of life, your sense of inner peace.

Corporations use a term called ROI, or return on investment, to assess the yield from an investment. In this case, you want to be able to assess the return on your investment in your health. When you are calculating your ROI, you need to measure the medical costs that you have saved, the insurance premiums that you have saved, the sick time from work that you have saved, the presenteeism in your workplace and the family life that you have eliminated in favor of active healthy participation. You can chart this over a month and then sequentially over a year and review on a year to year basis.

I recently received a letter from a study group member of our National Center for Homeopathy which clearly illustrates this point. She wrote, "Fifteen months after I began study with a study group, I had to collect my medical expense records for income tax purposes. Usually, I get a few hundred dollars over the 7.5% of adjusted gross income to deduct. For this past year, I had a few hundred dollars total, mostly for my daughter's insect bite and routine checkups. Discontinuing some prescription drugs and enjoying better health through homeopathy meant no tax deduction last year, because my total spent was way too low!"

As your health changes, so will the areas of investment. Note also what types of improvements have taken place in terms of energy, functionality, and effective relationships. Evaluate your ability to be creative and flexible in life situations as compared to prior years of investing in your health. Your ability to make changes, to move into uncharted territories and to leave behind strategies and relationships that are not adding value to your health are all signs of a growing economy within you. This is called resiliency. These are also signs of returns on your investment. The rate of return will always go up as a result of a sound investment in your health. When there are significant losses, it means it is time to reconfigure your portfolio. Sell off the investments that aren't performing and re allocate your assets. Invest your stress in areas that make it work for you, yielding high dividends on a daily basis. Stress that creates loss is a drag on profits. Cut the wasteful spending and invest in creating freedom, choice and autocracy.

Once you have identified your personal risk factors by going within and learning the language of yourself, you can design your own recession proof strategies as you develop an ideal investment portfolio, create long term wellness models, maximize dividends, experience a personal sense of satisfaction and celebrate the sensation of peace in your life.

As you practice this awareness, you become a perfect investor in your own business. You recognize feelings that will *not* yield dividends in accordance with your short term or long term strategies. Feelings of lack and incompetence will prompt you to make short term investments in daily activities such as meditation, stillness, mindfulness and the body/mind mapping activities that bring you insight into your present reality and allow you to access your strengths (assets). These you will invest for the long term.

PERFECT ASSET ALLOCATION

I love to use this word "perfect" because it evokes an immediate visceral response. Visceral means that you *feel* the emotion of perfection in your organs. Where do you feel it in your body when you hear the words "perfect asset allocation''? What are the thoughts and emotions that are evoked? Go back to your quiet space in your mind and check out the body map. The word *perfect* is fraught with emotions. Good emotions and not so good emotions. To some, perfect is a laudable goal. It breeds ambition at its best. Personal achievement. The thrill of winning. The feeling of a job well done. To others, it signifies a task too insurmountable to achieve. Perfect can bring out the horrors of low self esteem. Perfect can make one immediately retreat into a frozen mode of inaction. It is often difficult, if not impossible, even to begin a task if the word *perfect* is anywhere in the sentence.

The good news is that there is no perfect asset allocation. There is *optimal* asset allocation, however. That means that we do not have to worry about getting our asset allocation *perfect*. We can take our time to assess our strengths and weaknesses. We can develop our Health & Harmony Wellness Investment Portfolio over time. It is a process of learning who we are and watching how the landscape of our lives affects us. Our awareness of this tells us where our strengths and weaknesses lie.

Perfection is a dynamic process so one needn't worry if you do not appear perfect in the moment. The process is about refining our allocations all the time, throughout our lives. That being said, we can consider ourselves perfect in each moment! An attitude like this allows us to eliminate resistance to the idea or belief that we can never achieve perfection. Allowing abundance is an art form that develops when we stay in alignment with our Source energy and use our feelings to remind us of where we are in relation to Source on our way to wholeness.

HEALTH & HARMONY WELLNESS INVESTMENT PORTFOLIO

The circle is a symbol of the process that is at once complete in itself as there is no beginning and there is no end. Wherever you start, there you are!

Draw a circle and divide it up like pieces in a pie. The pieces will represent the areas that you will invest in. The pieces will be larger or smaller depending on your individuality.

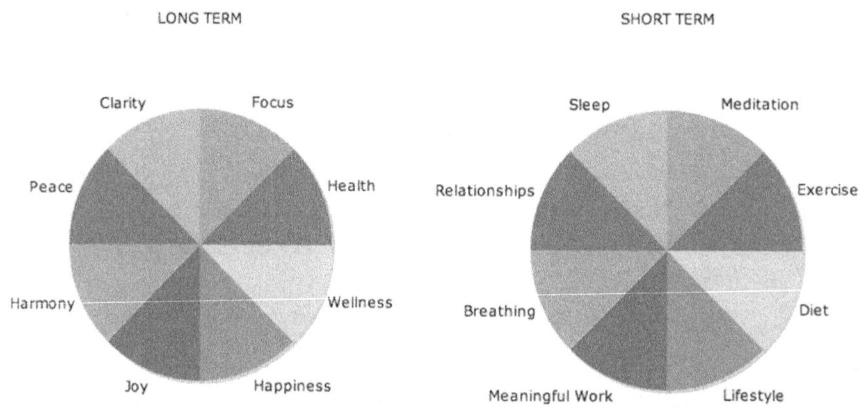

We invest so that we can reap the benefits of our hard work at some point when we are not able to work as hard. When we are young, we invest in more aggressive, risky allocations so as to yield higher dividends. As we age, we tend to conservative strategies that will preserve our capital investment and allow us to draw on these resources to use in our daily lives in our later years. The question at the outset is, what is your time horizon and your risk level?

In health terms, we have already come to understand these components from our work in Chapter 3. You have identified your emotional issues, the physical organs or systems that are primarily affected by the stressors that initiate illness and the language your Self speaks. The language and manifestation of symptoms are your liabilities. These are your risk factors. These may become chronic conditions and may require costly allopathic medical intervention. The older you are, the more likely this is. The younger you are, the more time you have to make short term investments that will eliminate these conditions and mitigate the need for, and expense of, long term chronic care.

Your assets are your strong points in body, mind, emotions and spirit. You have already determined where you are most healthy. You know your point of balance. You know where Home is. These are the considerations when you invest in short term, high yield strategies to grow your assets. Investing in areas such as meditation to stay clear and focused; exercise and proper eating to create health and energy; adequate sleep to promote refreshment and restoration of function; nurturing relationships to give meaning to your life; and doing work that stems from Source providing a service to the world will increase your daily dividends and create long term revenue in terms of health & harmony.

The key is to diversify. Proper asset allocation can prevent huge fluctuations in health returns and put you on the path to long term quality of life and growth.

Understanding your needs and making the appropriate wellness decisions to create a workable Health and Harmony Wellness Portfolio will provide you choice, freedom and flexibility in your lifetime to pursue all your goals and realize your dreams.

Each asset has its own cycle, so it is important to have different asset classes that are counter cyclical to each other so that your portfolio is balanced and has low volatility. A key concept is to diversify with different asset classes and to rebalance the portfolio in order to capture the opportunities of the time and manage the risks.

In the investment world, market timing is used to predict the asset class for this cycle. In our personal world we can do the same by identifying the cycle of life that we are in and make cogent predictions.

Young Woman - Age 17	
Long Term	**Short Term**
Homeopathic Consultations and Remedies	Meditation
	Stress Reduction
	Nutrition
	Yoga
	Exercise

Example 1: A young woman who suffers from premenstrual pain and moodiness can predict that she may likely suffer from hormonal issues through life cycles such as pregnancy, childbirth, perimenopause and menopause. In this case, she may want to invest long term in a constitutional homeopathic remedy that addresses her totality. She will likewise invest short term in supportive lifestyle classes such as meditation, nutrition, yoga, exercise. Market timing is a great tool to use when you are clearly in a cycle that has a predictable process or end point. This can be age related and so portends a timeline. Or it can be condition related that has a treatment protocol with a timeline.

The Talmud, the book of ancient Jewish law, (circa 1200BC-500AD), states "Let every man divide his money into three parts and invest a third in land, a third in business and a third let him keep in reserve."

We can apply this concept to the body/mind/spirit analogy. We can invest in land, our body; mind, our business and keep our reserves in spiritual escrow. Here we can go back to Chapter 3 and re-member who you are and where Home is. This is your reserve fund. Always keep it replenished, for here is where you draw upon to sustain yourself in the times when the market of your life takes a downturn.

Where is your reserve? How much do you have? Do you know how to keep that healthy?

CHAPTER 5

CREATING THE HEALTH & HARMONY WELLNESS INVESTMENT PORTFOLIO

Start from the beginning, zero, infinity, eternity. Formulate fresh decisions based on present position and future needs unencumbered by past decisions or limiting belief systems. Be an objective observer of your life and the way in which you envision it to become.

Never make decisions based on fear. Always make decisions based on power. In Chapter 3 you identified your issues. In Chapter 4 you learned how to use your assets to create your company... YOU. When you know how your assets are created, you never have fear because you always know how to create more.

Fear is an illusion. The opposite of what is real. Whenever you feel fear creeping into your thoughts, use this acronym. I believe it is attributable to Jack Canfield.

FEAR

False
Evidence
Appearing
Real

One belief system to identify and then disregard is a typical one that first time investors may fall prey to. One may understand that diversification reduces volatility, but simultaneously there exists the belief that diversification may limit returns. They feel that they may be spread too thin. Human nature tends to desire to put all their eggs in one basket and wait for the biggest omelet they have ever eaten! In reality, it is better to keep the eggs in different locations on the farm in case the fox gets at them or you trip and fall while carrying that big basket.

You can't be spread too thin if you appropriately identify your assets (and you will have more than one) and put them into different classes which are invested equitably. Equity investing keeps the long term in mind. We plan on being alive for approximately 70-80 years. It is tempting to watch for the immediate returns on an investment and abandon the long term strategies. This is especially true for the young as old age seems a long way off. My advice is to always devise and implement strategies with the long term in mind.

Conventional healthcare consists of allopathic medicine. That is, traditional medicine as we know it. The use of pharmaceuticals and surgery makes up this area. People with chronic conditions that would not be amenable to alternatives need to invest in this area according to their condition.

Chronic Conditions: Diabetes	
Long Term	**Short Term**
Allopathic Medecine	Nutrition
Health Insurance Program	Stress Management
Insurance Copayments	Exercise
Related Medical Expenses	Gym Membership
Homeopathic Consultations and Remedies	Yoga and Meditation Classes
	Socialization
	Support Groups

Example 2: If you have diabetes and are insulin dependent, that is not going to change. You must invest long term in allopathic medicine. That means that you must purchase a health insurance policy that will cover doctor visits, lab tests, prescriptions and home supplies for testing your blood sugar. The premium for that health insurance policy becomes part of your portfolio. Interestingly, diabetes is also a condition that is largely a self care condition. The majority of people with diabetes manage their care themselves with self testing, self medicating or injecting and managing their diet,exercise and stress. These are the areas of short term investments. The dollars that you spend on testing equipment and injectibles that are not covered by your insurance, as well as money spent on nutritional guidance, personal trainer, gym membership and yoga and meditation classes,become part of your short term investment profile and can be paid for through a qualified Health Savings Account or equivalent, if applicable in your State.

Evaluation of your diet and nutritional status is also a short term investment. Depending on several factors, one might use the library, Internet or local hospital Social Services to obtain information on your particular condition. This will reduce your cash outlay. In some cases, the more professional services of a certified nutritionist is required to prepare a specific plan for your individual needs. Factor these costs into your investment plan. Exercise figures prominently in the short term and long term of nearly e very disease process. Explore areas of exercise that you really like, feel good doing and, perhaps sharing with someone or participating in it as a hobby. There are walking,hiking and biking clubs as well as gyms that offer structured classes. Socializing often makes exercise more fun and motivates you to begin and to stick with it.

For those who do not require the socialization, cable networks have a vast array of shows to watch at home from yoga to tai chi to more strenuous exercise programs.

I would add to the portfolio, an investment in the services of a professional homeopath to consult with for constitutional treatment which strengthens your Self, stimulates the body to heal itself and enhances the effectiveness of the medicine you take. In some cases, patients report that they require less insulin when taking a homeopathic remedy suited for them. This is a cost savings and a good asset allocation.

Creating a Health & Harmony Wellness Investment Portfolio for a condition that you already have, such as the example of diabetes above, is one way of investing for your future when you know what you are dealing with.

How do you invest for your future when you do not have a disease or a condition that requires treatment?

You must challenge your beliefs in the sickness model of health-care and invest in prevention, wellness and health promotion.

The same principles apply when investing money in the stock market. We don't make investments predicated upon the belief that we will be impoverished at some point and will have to use all our money for sustenance . We take a look at our assets and liabilities (our strengths and weaknesses in health terms, our constitution), our present state of ability to earn an actual income (our state of health) and we make an assessment of what and how much we need to maintain our lifestyle financially. A projection of future needs is also taken into consideration. Then you invest for short and long term. The future is a given uncertainty and one thing that we can be sure of is that change happens. That is why you want to be fluid and flexible, agile, in your strategy and conservative or aggressive depending upon your character.

Young, Healthy Person	
Long Term	**Short Term**
Prevention and Health Promotion	Character Developments
Lifestyle	Healthy Relationships
No Smoking	Positive Attitude
Moderate Alcohol Consumption	Meaningful Work
Nutritionally Balanced Meals	Creating Happiness
Exercise	
Restorative Sleep	
Meditation and Mindfulness	
Stress Reduction Techniques	
Awareness and Avoidance of Environmental Pollutants and GMO Foods	

Example 3: A Health & Harmony Wellness Investment Portfolio for a young, healthy adult would be one where the long term investments are those that emphasize prevention, health promotion and wellness such as lifestyles that include not smoking, eating nutritious and well balanced meals, awareness and avoidance of environmental pollutants, periods of exercise and restorative sleep, meditation and mindfulness stress reduction techniques.

Short term investments are those that we can change with fluidity as needed such as relationships and jobs. Creating wellness is a function of development of character, self-reliance, confidence, courage and all the virtues that sustain us. These are gained through healthy, loving, supportive relationships. The attainment of happiness and a feeling of well being can yield dividends when one is gainfully employed in a job that is personally satisfying, in alignment with your Source and gives purpose to your life.

As one matures, relationships and jobs can be re-allocated as needed to ensure the best return on your investment.

Gracefully Aging Person: 50+	
Long Term	**Short Term**
Diet	Leisure Activities
Lifestyle Modifications	Healthy Relationships
Shorter Workdays	Job Assessment
Sleep Adjustments	Retirement Evaluation

Example 4: The gracefully aging person may have a Health & Harmony Wellness Investment Portfolio that has been yielding great returns as they have no diagnosable condition at their clinical horizon of 50 years old. It is generally assumed that what you have at 50 is a determinant for your future. If you have invested wisely in diet and lifestyle and have reached 50 relatively unscathed, then stay the course. Do not make any withdrawals. This is the time to invest more in the business of you that has been performing very well. Long term investments remain the same as to diet and lifestyle. Modifications due to age, such as shortening work days and increasing restorative rest, may well

be necessary but the formula stays the same. Keeping an eye toward retirement, you may want to look at where,how and with whom you will want to spend the next half of your life. Again, this requires that you go within and reassess your goals. Fulfilling your purpose in life and remaining in alignment with your Source continues until you transition from this life to the next. Hopefully, you will have it all down pat by then!

Golden Agers
Investments Yield Dividends
Live Your Best Life With The Assets You Have Accumulated

Example 5: Golden agers, who are relatively healthy, and there are some, specifically those who invested wisely, can take their profits and live the rest of their lives as they damn well please! Suze Orman, sage investment expert, advises that you spend your money while you are alive and not horde it to leave to your relatives when you die.

"Eat, drink and be merry, for tomorrow you may die!" I say live your best life through every age but certainly so in your last semester.

CHAPTER 6

WHERE DO I GO FROM HERE?

When you decide to look outside the box for "something else" this does require a few caveats. There is a collective term being used for those professions outside of allopathic or conventional medicine. It is called CAM, an acronym for Complementary and Alternative Medicine. The National Institute of Health (NIH) has a division called National Center for Complementary and Alternative Medicine (NCCAM). This center conducts research into those practices that are defined on their website so as to determine which ones are safe and effective and then they educate the public on their findings. See www.nccam.nih.gov. The budget is very limited and so the studies do not span the breadth of the safe and effective therapies that are currently practiced.

A more inclusive term is now being used, that is, integrative healthcare. Integrative healthcare emphasizes relationships. It emphasizes the individuality of each person and the need for the whole person to be addressed. Body, mind, emotion and spirit are in relationship to the function and sensation that make people responsive to others and to their environment. Integrative healthcare is a system that ensures that the whole person is taken into consideration when addressing their ills. Integrative healthcare acknowledges that relationship with other professionals is a must when coordinating the care of a whole person. Integrative healthcare brings the importance of social relationships, those of both family and community into consideration when evaluating a person's state of health or absence thereof.

Finding a place to start from, I advocate beginning with a review of the second largest system of medicine, homeopathy. Homeopathy is a whole system of medicine with its own medicines that are safe, gentle, non-toxic, effective and affordable. One of the beauties of homeopathy is that, because of the way in which the medicines are prepared, there are no adverse interactions with allopathic medicine. I tend to select this system of medicine as my first choice when working in an integrative way with other professionals and in the case of chronic disease management. The term Integrative Healthcare, as previously mentioned, is now the favored term for referencing practices outside of allopathic medicine.

It was generally agreed upon at the recent Institute of Medicine Summit on Integrative Medicine and the Health of the Public in Washington, D.C. that practices such as homeopathy are not complementary *nor* alternative but valid, stand alone systems of medicine that need to be perceived and referred to as such. Senator Harkins agreed and even said that he would change the name of NCCAM to the National Center for Integrative Healthcare. He acknowledged that, by eliminating the word "medicine," prejudice is removed and a single standard of care is eliminated in favor of choice of other systems.

I hold a vision of a world where there is choice and freedom within the healthcare system for us to choose the practitioner that best suits our needs. This vision is taking shape in our country as people are asking legislators to make laws that provide for non-discrimination among providers. The current version of healthcare reform, the Patient Protection and Affordable Care Act, which is now the law of the land, does contain language that includes a new category of the national healthcare workforce called "integrative healthcare practitioners". These are professions that are different from licensed doctors or nurses. They are a class of practitioners that hold national or state certifications that are accredited by the Institute for Credentialing

Excellence. They include Certified Classical Homeopaths (CCH) among other disciplines that offer diverse therapies that are as efficacious or more than allopathic medicine, without the side effects, and that generally cost less over time.

My goal in integrative healthcare is to connect with like-mided individuals in their pursuit of health and harmony, and invite them to focus their attention on the information, education, resources and the tools to set their Divine plan of self care into action.

When using the Internet to research choices, I advise that you look for professional organizations that have a standard of education or certification that indicates a level of proficiency within that profession. This does not mean a license, necessarily. The reason that a practice needs to be licensed, or regulated, is because it carries the threat of harm or danger. This is true for the practice of medicine. It is not true for the practice of homeopathy and that is why there is no license needed to practice homeopathy.

Homeopathy is safe for everyone to practice for self-limiting and many acute conditions. Complex, chronic conditions generally lend themselves to the efforts of a professional practitioner of homeopathy, often in concert with a doctor whose specialty is needed to work together effectively on a case. Many of these professionals, integrative healthcare practitioners, have studied extensively and may have received certification credentials from their organization. One example of this would be the letters CCH after one's name meaning Certified Classical Homeopath. These practitioners received this national credential from the Council for Homeopathic Certification. The CCH credential is available to all practitioners who meet the requirements and pass the examination whether they are licensed in another profession or not. A designated certification may be something that makes you feel comfortable when making a selection of a practitioner. For MD's or DO's, there is the Diplomat in Homeotherapeutics (DHt), for naturopaths,the certification is the DHANP, Diplomat of the Homeopathic Academy of Naturopathic Physicians.

For each profession in integrative healthcare that you are interested in, I suggest that you Google that name. There is usually a professional organization for that profession that will have a website with descriptions, resources and a practitioner base. For example, The National Center for Homeopathy (NCH) is the premier resource for information on homeopathy. The NCH is an open membership organization. You do not have to be a practitioner to join. Consumers join to receive information, webinars on home care, social media platforms to enjoy the camaraderie of like minded people and forums to share your experiences. And much more! Go to www.nationalcenterforhomeopathy.org to find out what homeopathy is and, more importantly, what homeopathy isn't. When you become a member of this organization, you become a valued person in the community at large with access to research, articles, webinars and events both online and in person. It is in the gathering of like-minded people that inspiration, enthusiasm and creativity is generated. Change is a result of the power of the people manifested in action.

Self care is largely a matter of using your resources to discover information about the choices available to you in your situation. People such as friends, neighbors, and relatives can be rich sources of information and are often happy to regale you with their stories of how they found their way. The incredible Internet is your other best friend. Be aware that some of the information available is not always accurate. You do need to check sources and cross check other sites. I think it is wise to go to Amazon.com and search for books on the subjects that you are interested in. Use those authors as references for your research. If they appear in related articles on the web, you have a better chance that the information is reliable.

Always, always, always, use your intuition. If it feels right, it is right. If it feels wrong, it is wrong.

ACCESS TO CHOICE

There is a new paradigm afoot largely due to the directive given to healthcare providers by President Obama. Wellness and prevention as a model for healthcare is the paradigm he is calling for. President Obama has called the medical/industrial complex to task for the spiraling costs of healthcare in a disease oriented system that does little to prevent the rising epidemic of chronic disease. He calls for personal responsibility on the part of each and every person.

A new paradigm calls for changes to or completely ousting the existing one. A reasonable approach to take is to keep what works and throw out the rest.

The best of conventional medicine appears to lie in its technological advances in surgery and truly therapeutic drugs. Truly therapeutic means those pharmaceuticals that are prepared with integrity of purpose. The purpose is to first, do no harm. Second, heal the person in the safest, gentlest way. The push to trivialize every symptom into a condition that has a jingle and a medication attached to it is one perversion of Big Pharma that is reprehensible to the public—and to many medical doctors as well. One recent study indicated that 50% of medical doctors were dissatisfied with the practice of medicine.

A well respected industry journal, The British Medical Journal (BMJ), recently reported that three quarters of all pharmaceutial research is written by Public Relations companies. The spin is what you see in advertisements.

Greed. The need to corner the market and have every person on one or more medications in their lifetime is the part of our medical system that must go.

The majority of stakeholders in the healthcare system agree that a new paradigm must include the person as the center of the system. Patient centered care or person centered care is one where the person plays an integral role in their care. People need to be educated in the basic concepts of wellness and prevention beginning with how to eat in a healthy manner, how to exercise for strength and endurance, how to manage life stresses to enhance immunity and how to create positive emotions to facilitate wellness and resilience. All the techniques that I spoke about earlier in this book are ones that every person must own so as to be competent partners in their healthcare with a well selected team of professionals.

Empowering people to self care will pave the way to wellness and prevention of chronic diseases. Self care starts at home. Before the advent of hospitals or the discovery of penicillin, sickness was handled at home. Women are the Original Primary Care Providers. From midwives to herbalists, the healing in families was traditionally through women. Mothers, in our day and age, still retain the intuition and wisdom to care for their families. Research shows that 85% of chronic diseases are preventable by diet and lifestyle. This fact puts healthcare, wellness and prevention squarely in the hands of the person in charge of shopping, cooking the meals and managing the daily activities of the family. We are in a time in our society where this role can be taken by the mother, the father or a designated provider. In my experience, it is predominantly the mother who calls the shots on the diet and lifestyle issues for the family. Access to healthy foods, modeling healthy behaviors and encouraging activities that are suitable for each member of the family is of paramount importance to achieving the quality of life that we all desire.

Creating the understanding that healthcare can be accessed in a retail food store where organic foods are sold is a paradigm shift from the understanding that one must seek "healthcare" when you are sick in a doctor's office. In my understanding, food IS medicine. Hippocrates, the fahter of medicine said, "Let food be your medicine and let medicine be your food". Our innate intelligence reminds us of this fact when we are "sick" and crave certain foods because they make us feel better. So called "old wives tales" are replete with recipes for curing ailments of all sorts. The most respected and well known cure for a common cold is chicken soup. I know that my particular recipe is the first line of defense whenever a sniffle or cough appears. My children ask for it when they are run down or under stress. I sent my son an overnight delivery of chicken soup this fall when he was away at college and "under the weather" from the stress of final examinations. Was it the organic ingredients, homegrown herbs, the intent or the love that cured him? We will never know the placebo effect of chicken soup but we all are aware of its healing capabilities. Access to healthcare, wellness and prevention is a matter of simple self care at home.

When foods are not enough to bring the body back into balance, we can look to individualize the treatment further using homeopathic remedies.

The best part of the new paradigm would be that one can purchase homeopathic remedies in retail stores. Thankfully, this is already the case. Forward thinking retailers such as Whole Foods, Vitamin Shop, Duane Reade and others carry a line of homeopathic remedies for self care. Self care is effective for the majority of self-limiting conditions. Self- limiting conditions are those that would resolve without intervention in 3-7 days. Self care with homeopathic remedies affords quicker relief of suffering and a gentle return to better health. Astute consumers can treat themselves for the viral syndromes like a cold for which allopathy has no answer. Parents can treat their child who has an earache, or uncomplicated fever without running to the emergency room of an already overburdened hospital system. Women can treat themselves for the annoying to devastating disabling symptoms of perimenopause and menopause, another area where medicine has no answer. Simple sprains and strains, cuts and bruises, sunburns and bug bites can be effectively managed personally with homeopathic remedies.

The world I envision calls for premeditation. By determining what your constitution is, that is, where your strengths and weaknesses lie, you can prepare for emergencies in a better way. With aforethought, you can create a team of professionals, as we discussed, who are best suited to assist you with your short term healthcare goals as well as identifying those specialists whom you may need in the future given your inherent predispositions. The challenge of what to do and whom to turn to in a crisis situation then becomes a non-entity.

Empowering people to take responsibility for themselves is just what the *new* doctor ordered! This paradigm of health-care will drastically reduce the medical costs to our system, improve relationships in the home and workplace and thus, improve productivity overall which leads to....happiness! A fundamental marker of health and well-being.

With more responsibility, however, the economic burden is shifted back to you as well. Over the counter healthcare products, herbal, homeopathic, nutritional or even those such as Tylenol are not covered by insurance. Neither are the professional consultations of professional integrative healthcare practitioners. Nor are education, books, and seminars that are necessary to get you up to speed on self care, wellness and prevention.

While the prospects of healthcare going retail appear enticing, the truth is that many people will not understand how to allocate their expenses in this direction. To test this theory, I stood in a retail store that carried homeopathic medicines during the flu season. There was a dizzying array of cough, cold and flu products to choose from. I saw the perplexed look on the faces of people as they read the ingredients on the "natural" products. *Which to choose?* It was clear that they wanted something natural or homeopathic but were confounded as to what helped what. One person asked the pharmacist about the homeopathic product that she was holding, alas, to no avail. He was a pharmacist, after all, not a homeopath. So, the person left the package on the counter and walked out. Another person asked the sales clerk which cough preparation she would use, a combination homeopathic one or Robitussin. She was advised to take the Robitussin.

I brought this question up for discussion in my homeopathic study group on self care for Moms. *How would they make a selection?* One said she would choose what her mother had always given her or one whose name was familiar. I asked if she would choose a homeopathic remedy and she said that she would be hesitant because she didn't know what the ingredients were. Then I asked her if she knew what the ingredients were in Robitussin and how they worked and she admitted that she didn't but would feel safer with that because she knew it has been around for a long time. *Did it work?* That didn't seem to matter. *Was it safe?* Most astonishing was one person's perception that if it is sold in Duane Reade then it is safe *and* effective!

An article in Oprah magazine, June, 2009 titled, "Drug Deception" confirms this fact. "People tend to assume that if a drug is available in the U.S., it is safe and it works," said Amy Allina, program director of the National Women's Health Network. The fact is that thousands of drugs, prescription only, sold in pharmacies and even covered by insurance have never been approved by the U.S. Food and Drug Administration. The article goes on to say that "unapproved drugs exist in a sort of legal limbo." According to Patti Manolakis, a health policy consultant from Charlotte, North Carolina, "They have names and packaging that look just like the approved drugs, and they're even in the *Physicians' Desk Reference*." Many more drugs are used "off line" meaning that they have been approved for one condition but are being used for a totally different condition.

So, who do you trust? Trust yourself! Personal responsibility means that you are in charge of your own business. You, as CEO of yourself, are responsible for ferreting out the correct information, synthesizing it into what is best for you according to your Health and Harmony Wellness Investment Portfolio, and selecting the best products and services to meet your goals. The sage investor, Warren Buffet, when asked what he thought was the best investment strategy, replied, "Invest in yourself". His ROI's are significant! I advocate for his strategy which is mine as well.

Even though homeopathic remedies are available in retail stores, access to choice of homeopathic practitioners is another area that needs to be expanded upon. Similar to the current dilemma in medicine of having too few primary care physicians to serve the population, so it is with homeopathic practitioners. The profession is small in numbers but growing rapidly. The fact that homeopathic services are not reimbursed by insurance companies is an obstacle to many people who want to use their services but feel that they already pay so much for insurance premiums that they must use the physicians on their plan. Secondly, because of the high insurance premiums, people often do not have discretionary income available to use for homeopathic care.

The solution becomes easier to see when you look back at your Health and Harmony Wellness Investment Portfolio and discover the areas you need to invest in to yield the highest return. Return on Investment, ROI, is what you are striving for. That being said, when diversifying in health care services, some of your investment will be cash outlay for those services not covered by insurance. You will need to budget for that. The truth is that homeopathic care is very affordable compared to medical care. Cost comparison studies abound to attest to this fact. Homeopathy has been a primary care modality in Europe for 200 years with a track record to prove its effectiveness and affordability as well as patient satisfaction.

Initial consultations will have the highest cost. "Taking a case", as it is called in homeopathy requires approximately 2 hours. Time spent is dependent on complexity and chronicity of the case. Fees range from $150-200. an hour in metropolitan areas and can be less in rural areas. This is yet one more reason to be aware that an ounce of prevention is worth a pound of cure. When health issues are addressed when they are minor, there is less out of pocket expense. A simple visit to your homeopath when you are suffering symptoms of a virus will cost less than if you wait until you have a secondary bronchitis or complicated pneumonia. Let common sense prevail. Crisis intervention is a thing of the past medical model. Don't wait until your business is going into bankruptcy to look for a bail out. Address the minor symptoms in a timely manner and the big picture will take care of itself.

That said, follow up visits to a homeopath are determined by the nature and complexity of your condition. A plan will be discussed at the outset of your care and you can fit this into your yearly budget. Due to the dearth of practitioners and geographic factors, many homeopaths will do telephone consultations. The ever advancing technologies, such as Skype, FaceTime and iChat, allow us the pleasure of face-to-face communication. The time saved and travel costs saved can actually pay for the visit. My telehealthcare service, TeleHealthandHarmony is very easy to use via Internet and receives accolades due to the time saved both in travel and lost hours from work or family responsibilities as well as the quick response to early treatment via information prescriptions.

Recently, I was away on vacation in Mexico. While I had promised my husband that I wouldn't do any work, I did sneak a look at my iPad while he was in the restroom. There was a message from a dear friend and patient of mine who was suffering from sciatica. She wanted an appointment. I responded that I was on vacation but would see her upon my return. When I gave her that date, she replied that she couldn't make that appointment time as she had an appointment with her dermatologist for an "unrelated" rash on her back. A light bulb went off and I asked her to send me a picture of the rash. Within minutes my suspicion was confirmed. She had a case of shingles. The sciatic nerve root was affected. I told her to keep her dermatologist appointment, gave her an information prescription for a homeopathic remedy to ease the pain and stimulate healing and an appointment to follow up with me upon my return for chiropractic care of the sciatica.

In a matter of 10 minutes, this patient received a diagnosis and a treatment plan and peace of mind over the weekend while waiting to see her doctor. The cost was $50. No insurance. No middle man. Simplicity and peace of mind.

I encourage everyone to partake of telehealthcare in instances where it is not an emergency or life threatening sitution.

Inquire at askdrnancy@aol.com for further information and consultation.

Cost effectiveness is enhanced with homeopathic care because of its self care nature. You become directly involved in the experience of your healing and therefore, it is the most rapid and gentle way to return to health. The healthier you are, the less money it costs to maintain that state. The more present and informed you are about your own health, the more you can care for yourself. The need for professional intervention then becomes a quarterly check up, perhaps. I like to have my patients check in at every change of season. A fee of $75. four times a year is $300. for general maintenance. You can budget that in to your yearly expenses so you are prepared for that amount of expenditure each year. You also view it as an investment in your long term health. A common human desire is to have control over our lives. It is the desire of every person who has come to me for care to feel a sense of inner peace, to be free from physical pain and to have all their dreams come true. This way of thinking and acting in your own best interest is one of the best ways I know of to engender that feeling of being in control of your life.

CHAPTER 7

THE LONG ROAD HOME

So we find ourselves back at the place where we began. Home.

Health, wellness, prevention, happiness—they all begin at home. I do favor self care. I do favor home centered care. I do favor an integrative approach to healthcare with the person at the center. I do favor a system that offers choice and access to other practices and medicines.

I also favor a change in the way in which these services and products are reimbursed. It is no secret that insurance is here to stay. It appears, at this point in the conversation, that you can be reasonably certain that benefits will be determined by a medical standard of care. That means that the choices we have discussed will not be covered by insurance.

Back to the same point, again and again. Personal responsibility means that you advocate for what you want. Change and access to choice comes about by persistence.

At this juncture, I believe that change will come about by a revolution. Consumers must demand what they want. A wellness revolution is long past due!

We need to advocate for reimbursement for the practitioner services and products of your choice, including those carried in the retail food stores. Maybe even organic foods should be reimbursable or tax deductible. Well, that may be a stretch right now, but we are dealing in future commodities here. We are making long term investments in our Health and Harmony

Wellness Portfolio, and we surely know that diet plays a key role in disease and its prevention. Further, we are certain that pesticides are toxic and genetically modified (GMO) foods are dubious at best.

Creating a new paradigm means making changes. Changes we can all believe in. Change doesn't happen overnight. Changes of this matter require constant vigilance and the cooperation of all parties involved. The change agents in this case are your legislators. Call them, write to them, visit their local offices and tell them what you want. Tell them that you want choice in your healthcare of other systems of medicine and healing, integrative practices. Tell them that you want access to integrative healthcare practitioners of your choice. Tell them that you want choice in your insurance plan. Tell them that you want health savings accounts that allow for payment of wellness consultations, homeopathic remedies, vitamins, supplements, massage, stress management, Reiki, chiropractic, meditation and the like. These are some of the services that are safe, effective, non-toxic, and that enhance wellness and prevent disease. These and others like them are the services that you would like to invest in. Tell them that you would like to invest your Health and Harmony Wellness Portfolio in a money market instrument that avails itself of tax exemptions in a health savings accounts. All that needs to be done is to change the language for inclusion. Sen. Orrin Hatch is sponsoring a bill at present to expand the language. The bill is S.1098, Title: Family and Retirement Health Investment Act. Call his office. Write to him and support this bill.

Health savings accounts were created to relieve the burden of expensive medical care and to allow people the freedom to choose the practitioner, products and services of their choice. Again, the only choices available at present are medical doctors and medical services. The one prevailing standard of care is allopathic medicine. In my understanding, this is called a monopoly. This is what needs to be changed. This requires a change in the language of the existing bill, as mentioned. Pat Rooney is the innovative thinker and creator of the concept of health savings accounts to give power back to the consumer. He has written a wonderful, informative book on this subject that I highly recommend you read. *America's Health care Crisis Solved by J. Patrick Rooney and Dan Perrin.* Knowledge is power. You certainly want to be well informed when you advocate on behalf of yourself. Know what you want, then ask for it. Then persist. Persistence and you never fail is an adage worth remembering.

Another adage worth remembering is from one of our founding fathers, Thomas Jefferson. He said, " The price of freedom is eternal vigilance".

While you are asking, make a case for health freedom legislation on a state by state basis. Health freedom legislation protects those people using practices other than allopathic medicine from being accused of practicing medicine without a license. The National Health Freedom Coalition is the resource for current information on this very important topic. Visit their website at http:/www.nationalhealthfreedomcoalition.org

Choice. Change. That change that we can believe in. It is all a matter of asking for what you want and staying on message. It is work. It may seem easier to accept the status quo or to let someone else do the grunt work. Look around you. Is the status quo serving your best interest? Have you seen a viable return on your investment? Is the business of being you thriving? Have the other people that you put in charge been doing their best for you?

Personal responsibility and self care means that you are in charge of yourself. My husband is fond of saying, "If it is going to be, it is going to be because of me."

It may seem like a long way home from here, but put one step in front of the other, actualize all the principles I've taught you, believe in yourself and before you know it, there you will be! There is no place like Home!

RESOURCES

Health & Harmony Wellness Education

www.drnancygahles.com

The National Center for Homeopathy

www.nationalcenterforhomeopathy.org

National Health Freedom Coalition

www.nationalhealthfreedomcoalition.org

Washington Homeopathic

www.homeopathyworks.com

Homeopathic Educational Services

www.homeopathic.org

REFERENCES

Besant, Annie. Wisdom.

Bible, The Holy.

British Medical Journal, The.

Deng-Ming-Dao. 365 Tao:Daily Meditations. July 17,1992.

Dyer, Wayne. Change Your Thoughts, Change Your Life:Living The Wisdom of the Tao. Hay House, 2009.

Emerson, Ralph Waldo. Self-Reliance. 1841.

Grimm, the Brothers. Hansel and Gretel. 1979.

Hahnemann, Samuel,M.D. Organon of the Medical Art. 1842.

Hill, Napolean. Think and Grow Rich. Penguin Books, 2005.

Institute of Medicine of the National Academies. Summit on Integrative Medicine and the Health of the Public. Feb. 27, 2009.

Isaacson, Walter. Einstein, His Life and Universe.bSimon and Schuster. 2007.

Klotz, Neil Douglas. Original Prayer. Sounds True. www.soundstrue.com.

Lansky, Amy. Impossible Cure, The Promise of Homeopathy. R.L. Ranch Press. 2003.

Lansky, Amy. Active Consciousness. Awakening The Power Within. R.L. Ranch Press. 2011.

Lao Tzu. Tao Te Ching. Penguin Classics. 1963.

McTaggart, Lynne. The Field. The Quest for the Secret Force of the Universe. Harper. 2008.

Montagnier, Luc. New Scientist. Andy Coughlin. 12 Jan. 2011.

National Center for Complementary and Alternative Medicine. www.ncam.nih.gov.

National Center for Homeopathy. www.nationalcenterforhomeopathy.org

National Health Freedom Coalition. www.nationalhealthfreedomcoalition.org.

Oprah Magazine. Drug Deception. June, 2009.

Pert, Candace B., Ph.D. Molecules of Emotion. Scribner. 1997.

Price, John Randolph. The Jesus Code. Hay House. 2000.

Rooney, J. Patrick and Dan Perrin. America's Healthcare Crisis Solved. Wiley. 2008.

Rush, Benjamin, M.D. Quotes.

Seuss, Theodor, Dr. Oh, the Places You'll Go! Random House. 1990.

Talmud.

Wizard of Oz. Film. 1939.

ABOUT THE AUTHOR

I shall be telling this with a sigh
Somewhere ages and ages hence:
Two roads diverged in a wood, and I-
I took the one less travelled by,
And that has made all the difference.
-Robert Frost

Dr. Nancy Gahles is a Doctor of Chiropractic (DC) in family practice for over 30 years in NY and NJ. She is a Certified Classical Homeopath (CCH) and President Emeritus of the National Center for Homeopathy.

Dr. Gahles' passion as an ardent patient advocate is channeled through her service as a member of the Board of Directors of the Integrative Healthcare Policy Consortium, where she also serves as Chair of the Federal Policy Committee. She is a member of the healthcare working group of the American Sustainable Business Council. She infuses the conversation with spirituality through her vocation of Ordained Interfaith Ministry and joyfully creates ceremonies of marriage, life transitions and end of life services.

Dr. Gahles is a free lance journalist and healthcare columnist.

She is a member of the Advisory Board for the Integrative Healthcare Symposium.

Through her writing, lecturing, teaching, practicing, mentoring and advocating, Dr. Gahles is an internationally recognized expert in the field of integrative healthcare.

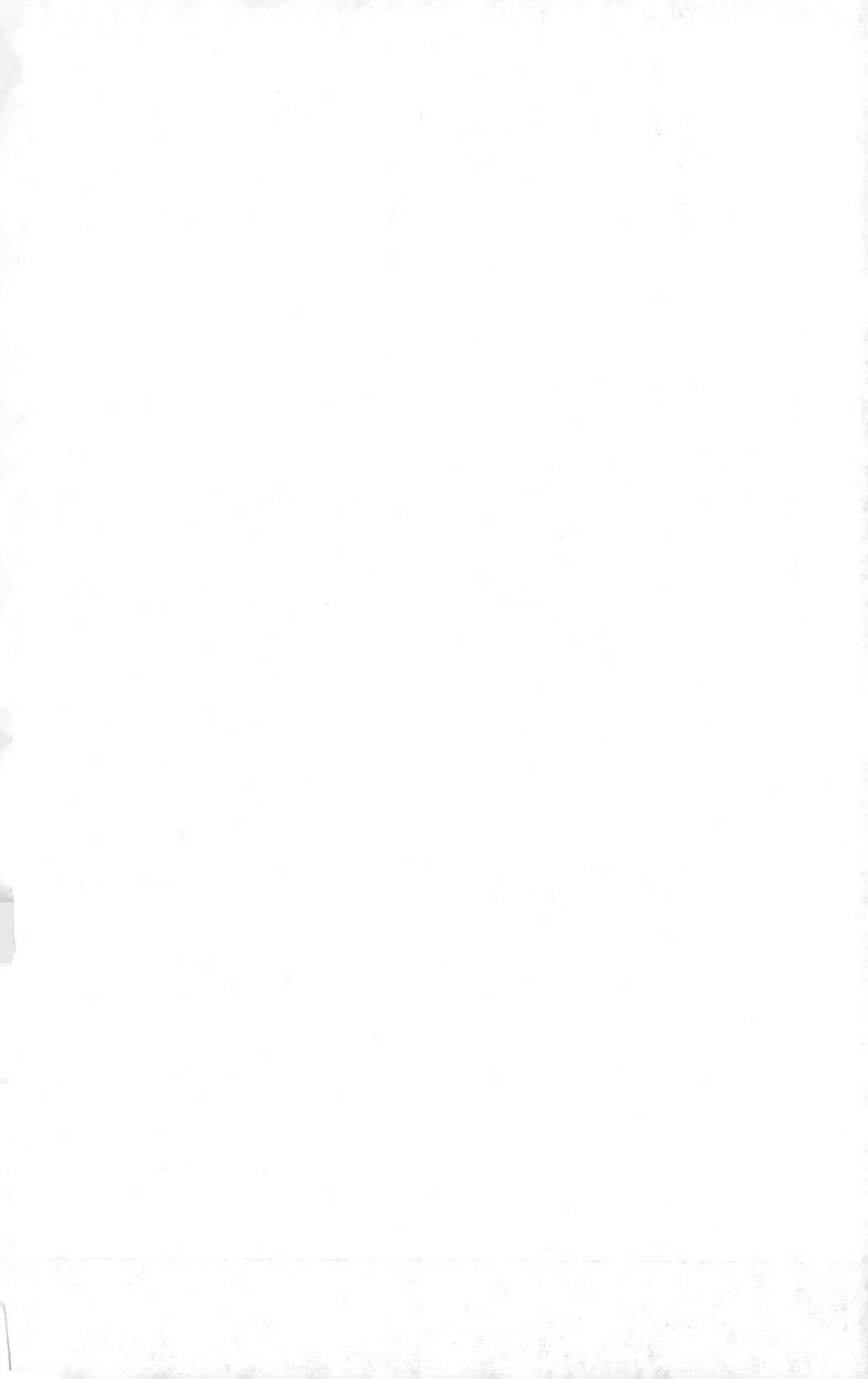

www.ingramcontent.com/pod-product-compliance
Lightning Source LLC
Chambersburg PA
CBHW060152290526
45789CB00003B/1013

9781470013783